PRESCRIBING FAITH

PRESCRIBING FAITH
Medicine, Media, and Religion
in American Culture

Claire Hoertz Badaracco

BAYLOR UNIVERSITY PRESS

Cover Design by Pamela Poll
Cover image: Nineteenth-century pharmaceutical trade cards. Courtesy of
the Newberry Library, Wing Collection Foundation.

Library of Congress Cataloging-in-Publication Data

Badaracco, Claire.
  Prescribing faith : medicine, media, and religion in American culture /
Claire Hoertz Badaracco.
      p. cm.
  Includes bibliographical references and index.
  ISBN 978-1-932792-89-8 (alk. paper)
  1. Medicine—Religious aspects. 2. Alternative medicine—United States—
History. 3. Spiritual healing—United States—History. 4. Mass media—
Religious aspects. 5. Health in mass media. I. Title.

  BL65.M4B33 2007
  201'.6610973—dc22

                                                          2007026451

Printed in the United States of America on acid-free paper with a minimum
of 30% pcw recycled content.

To the readers' good health!

CONTENTS

ACKNOWLEDGMENTS

The contributions of interdisciplinary research and archival experts made this book possible. I want to thank Dr. Paul Gehl, Curator of the Wing Foundation Collection on the History of Printing at the Newberry, for his interest in my research and his friendship for more than a decade. I also want to thank Honor Hill, Judy Huenecke, Michael Davis, Jonathan Eder, and the archival staff of the Eddy Collection. Thanks also to the staff in the Rare Book Room of the Countway Library of Harvard Medical School, and to Dr. Stephen Greeenberg of the National Library of Medicine and Arlene Shaner at the New York Academy of Medicine, and to the Berg Collection of the New York Public Library.

I wish to extend my thanks to my dean, Dr. John Pauly, at Marquette University, Deiderich College of Communication, where I am a Professor teaching media and religion. Thanks also to the Mary Baker Eddy Foundation for the Betterment of Humanity, and to the Newberry Library Consortium, all of which provided small grants in support of this research. The views expressed in this book do not represent those of any contributors, nor do they intend to represent the views of any religious denomination.

I especially want to thank the intellectual leaders of the field of Media, Religion, and Culture, especially Dr. Stewart Hoover at the University of Colorado Center for the Study of Media, Religion, and Culture, from whom I have learned so much over the past ten years. Thanks also for his leadership in the field to Dr. John Ferre of the University of Louisville, and to the many other scholars who have advanced the body of knowledge in the field of culture, media, and religion in significant ways.

A special word of thanks is due to Dr. Carey Newman, Diane Smith, and to the Baylor University Press editorial staff, whose attention to the finer points of producing a volume of distinction are highly valued and so greatly appreciated.

FIGURES

INTRODUCTION

Protect us from all anxiety, as we wait in joyful hope . . .

—ancient Latin prayer

At a time in our cultural history when monks and poets say anxiety is an American pandemic, and the pharmaceutical sector reaps more profits than oil, the fastest-growing popular medicine movement is emerging from what the National Institutes of Health (NIH) term "complementary and alternative medicine." One aspect of the complementary and alternative medicine movement is mind-body medicine, within which prayer is one among many therapeutical approaches to healing, including Eastern meditative practices employed in stress reduction among those with cardiovascular disease. The pluralistic approaches to medicine, including the ancient prayers of many faiths, and contemplative science, along with ethnic, folk, and botanical cures, have gained so much credence among Americans that over the first five years in the twenty-first century more people used National Center for Complementary and Alternative Medicine (NCCAM) practitioners than they did physicians, if NIH government statistics are accurate.

According to the NCCAM at the National Institutes of Health, the practice of complementary and alternative medicine consists of many

1

elements, including approaches to a sustainable environment, and botanical, biological, neurological, religious, and spiritual approaches to healing and to health. Some of these concepts are centuries old, some integrate Western with Eastern approaches to healing, and some use plants as cures. Yet doctors warn against the toxicity of natural and herbal cures at the same time that the pharmaceutical industry spends billions in research and development for new drugs and millions more

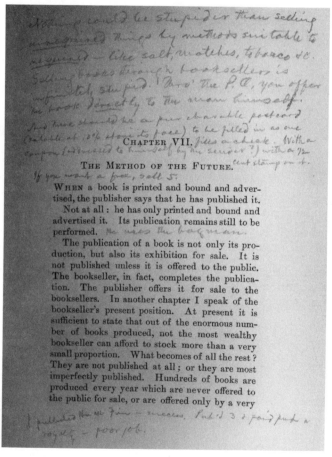

Figure 0.1: "The Method of the Future." *Mark Twain's marginalia on Sir William Besant's* The Pen and The Book (*London: Thomas Burleigh, 1899*). *Courtesy of the Newberry Library, Wing Collection Foundation on the History of Printing.*

in advertising them; some of these have proven fatal while still under patent protection.

Among the mix of controversial cures about medicine and healing today, none are more controversial than the role of faith, particularly if prescribed as part of a therapeutic culture in which advertising disease thrives. The purpose of this book is to explore the historical roots of that controversy and, as the final chapter asserts, to deconstruct the pseudoscience of disease awareness that creates a demand for anxiety as a product, one that requires the corollary production of faith-based products to alleviate fears of illness, aging, and death. Yet the evidence seems to demonstrate that there are two sectors of the American economy of health: the rejectors of standard medicine and those who buy in. As the question of healing becomes increasingly polarized, the fence-sitters or "undecideds" are decreasing.

According to the economic theory of rational choice, especially as it has been applied to religion, when the surplus of similar goods increases, there is a greater need for branding, the cultural storytelling that creates differentiation in the mind of the consumer. The greater the number of choices, the deeper the loyalties among those who prefer one cure over another. According to the theories of publicity, wherever there is a polarized public, loyalties deepen in their allegiance to their choice, and as a result the opposition has no credibility. Where credibility is lacking, so is trust. Wherever there is a lack of trust, advertising exacerbates disbelief. The more involved marketers get in selling drugs to the already anxious and fearful American public, the less trust they have for the medical establishment. As history demonstrates, medical and religious authority once were mixed, and as medicine professionalized, doctors tried to distance themselves in the twentieth century from the irrational beliefs of the clergy in the nineteenth. "Take it on faith," then, can apply to the prescriptions of the contemporary pharmaceutical culture, as it once did to the toxic cures of nineteenth-century physicians.

What is it about American cultural identity that has cultivated the ground for alternative religions based on the rejection of formal medicine and its prescriptions? Why did these "alternative" ideas about medicine and religious healing become so popular? Are they endemic to the American culture? Shouldn't the advances in science that occurred by the twenty-first century preclude such "irrational" choice? What drives social movements based on therapeutic beliefs? Are they constructions of media? Are they fads that will peak and fade in due course? Not so, this book asserts—they are part of American culture and its engrained ambivalence toward religion and health, rooted not only in popular beliefs and fads and tipping points, but also in the deeper levels of our cultural heritage, in literary culture, in the history of the book, in women's history, and in the ways in which both medicine and religion are in the business of advertising hope.

In complementary and alternative medicine, within which mind-body medicine is the most frequently practiced, the fields of cognitive psychology, positive thinking, neuroscience, Buddhist mental training, and Christian prayers for healing converge. The contrarian force is economic: the power of the global pharmaceutical industry, or "Big Pharma," disseminated into the popular culture through the mass media using the method of branded advertising—selling the drugstore as habitus, in unbranded, disease condition advertising, called "disease mongering," or in the news industry that foments anxiety about epidemics based on science drawn from press releases written by public relations agents. The media covers science as news, but research shows that very few journalists are trained with an adequate science education to unpack the research behind the press releases; a host of social forces behind the media reports thus escape the reporter and bypass their audience.

While "not everyone can pray," as William James observed, everyone can imagine, and everyone can worry. In fact, the imagination of disease is at the heart of the new science of advertising illness in order to sell pharmaceuticals as a universal panacea that is a product with spiritual content, in the sense that it advocates a certain position about where to put one's faith, where value lies in the healing of the body. In a converged economy, electronic news, Internet information, and advertising and public relations are all tying together the role of rational choice by consumers to the hope of wellness into a cultural vocabulary that transcends ethnicity or denomination, and reincarnates historically entrenched ideas about medicine, wellness and faith.

The historical search for a healing presence in American culture is mirrored in and sustained by today's mass media. As a case in point, consider the cover of *Newsweek* magazine from November 10, 2003, one that posed the archetypal question for the twenty-first century, "God and Health: Is Religion Good Medicine? Why Science is Starting to Believe." In other words, can believing make a difference in physical health? Though many doctors today still are reluctant to talk about faith with their patients, some are attempting to measure the impact of belief on healing, and faith on health. The *Newsweek* headline pointed to the issue's feature article, about a physician's research in the healing power of faith. Yet the cover image was not a doctor, but a woman patient depicted in a prayer of supplication, we presume, awaiting the ministrations of a doctor, in whom she must put her faith. In media marketing, the more universal the image, the better the magazine's chances of hooking an audience, of getting readers to see themselves in the scenario on the cover. Both magazines and advertising use similar methods to reach mass audiences, and the same global advertising and public relations firm might hypothetically employ both the media buyer who places an advertisement for a pharmaceutical company and an international marketer responsible for promoting a newsmagazine. The image on the cover of *Newsweek* was of a woman in a green patient's gown sitting in her hospital bed, manicured hands, clear polish, no wedding ring, with the hospital's plastic identity bracelet on her right arm. She looked up toward the "light" of the blue background at the top of the page as the print paled above the magazine title. Her psycho-demographic profile would be described this way: young, white, of child-bearing years, college educated, lives in the suburbs of a major metropolitan area, exercises regularly, eats well, doesn't smoke, and thinks positively about her future. Possibly the cover's "every woman" is like the reader who also subscribes to *Elle* or *Vogue* or *Bazaar* or *Women's Wear*, and if she does flip through those pages while waiting for her doctor's appointment, she will encounter there a similar mirroring effect, a refrain of repetitive images in the advertisements in those pages filled with as many beauty tips for antiaging face creams as pharmaceutical advertisements related to women's health.

Historically, popular knowledge about natural health and the body's ability to heal itself has existed in a contested space, constructed in opposition to doctors' prescriptions and the ideas about "regular medicine" that have shaped healing practices in American medical education and the established infrastructure of research and clinical trials. It remains a contested space today, but the players have changed, now including the global monolithic power of the pharmaceutical industry and the science of public opinion engineering.

Given the impact of mass media on the social economy of medicine, the central inquiry of this book is about how media will converge with the role of religion, faith, belief, and spirituality, and what effect that will have on the type of care readers expect, especially if they enter a hospital. Will they expect to have the admitting department take their spiritual history along with their medical one? Will it free them to talk with their doctors about religion? Then will they talk with their pastor about science questions? In turn, will the clergy feel authorized to talk about science from the pulpit, particularly if that science question is loaded with political or public policy freight, and if they do, will that violate the tax laws of the U.S. government's Internal Revenue Service?

Some argue that all this convergence is not only bad for medicine, it is bad for religion. The news media is not among those that argue this point, however, for they seem to come at it fresh, as if there were no historical memory of debates, which have been going on in America for the past century. Religion in the practice of medicine remains among the most controversial subjects in medical literature today, and one can understand why.

As this book discusses, the mediated public debate about science and religion is communicated today through three interrelated threads: (1) impact of prayer on health, (2) intelligent design vs. creationism, and (3) national health-care public policy and constitutional or Supreme Court jurisprudence issues such as *Roe v. Wade*. This book unpacks the first of those threads, and by doing so provides a platform to understand better the public conversation about medicine and religion, within its historical frame, and clarify the tension between current medical practices and the trend toward alternative and complementary medicine, within which flourish the ideas about the healing power of faith.

This book frames the discussion of the subject by the historically significant episodes revealed by the currents in both American religion and medicine, the belief and the imagination, and how the two are intertwined. It is about how the power of medical belief shaped Romanticism during the Transcendentalist era in the nineteenth century. The power of disbelief in heroic cures that defined the Romantic's search for a natural religion in Transcendentalism during the era of the rise of the medical establishment at Harvard shifted at the turn of the twentieth century, from reliance on heroic prescriptions, medicines so toxic that they tested patients' courage, to reliance on biblical interpretation, and intuitive or "inspired" knowledge postulated as scientific. This shift at the turn of the century disengaged the popular gaze from the objective scientist to the subjective patient, and the controversy that ensued continues today but with constituents speaking in a new vocabulary of alternatives to medicine, reinventing the centuries-old language about the mind, psychology and the brain, neuroscience, and its influence on health.

Women play a key role in this history as both object and subject. It was the woman neurasthenic on whom early nineteenth-century doctors tested their toxic cures and to whom ministers preached about how good it was to suffer—how it formed character and how it pleased the Lord and bonded the sufferer to their progeny and domestic duties. Later, it was women pioneers—entrepreneurs if you like—such as Mary Baker Eddy who, with a strong determination wrought from deep suffering, decided that they preferred to be the heroines of their own lives rather than occupy an objective place in the formulations of medical doctors anxious to advance the state of medical knowledge and to claim it as their own.

In the first chapter, the lives of Sophia Peabody and her doctor, Walter Channing, offer a glimpse into the history of heroic cures and Transcendentalist thought about the purposes of suffering and how gender and physiology intersected with those ethereal beliefs. Medical advice books based on botanical cures were on the hearth of every home. The medical establishment was only beginning to be professionalized, and many patients thought about ministers and doctors as one and the same. Channing was in many ways a heroic character. A founder of Harvard Medical School, he wanted to help alleviate suffering among women in childbirth. But his life also contained elements of the tragic, as did Sophia's, who suffered under Channing's prescriptions of heroic cures of arsenic and mercury until she undertook a recuperative trip to Cuba. Suffering and the role of the patient in the construction of American medicine, and in the convergence of medical and spiritual authority, are illustrated by the episodes from the lives of these eminent Transcendentalists who lived in New England in the nineteenth century.

In the second chapter, the life of Mary Baker Eddy is profiled because she rejected what seemed so normal and acceptable to the genteel female invalids who typified the period. Eddy lived a long time, dying in 1910 at the age of ninety, and her biography has been well documented by more than seventy-five admirers and detractors, which the reader may wish to consult for a fuller picture of her fascinating life. Her full biography is beyond the scope of the purposes of this book; she is profiled as representative of a time in American religious culture in which medicine and healing converged, much as it does today. This chapter focuses on how Eddy used media, particularly the religious book. It is also a story about how a woman of such leadership could also be capable of human error. Yet it was her book, *Science and Health with Key to the Scriptures*, edited and revised nearly 250 times, that contributed to the market position of the religious book in the history of American publishing, one competitive with trade presses and news media.

Mark Twain—the humorist and cultural icon who wrote books, as well as articles for newspapers and magazines—on the surface an affable competitor, was capable of wicked satire while at the same time full of admiration for the person he satirized. This book's frontispiece, graciously contributed from the vault of the Newberry Library's Wing Foundation Collection on the History of Printing, is Twain's marginalia, scribbling in pencil on his personal library copy of Sir William Besant's *The Pen and the Book*, published in 1898. I selected this as the unifying image for this volume because it captures the moment, at the turn of the century, when branding entered all realms of high and low culture, from religion to books to medicine. Twain's marginal comments show him in agreement with the ideas in *The Pen and The Book* about modern selling. As my second chapter takes up, the archival evidence reveals Twain as obsessed by a comparison of his profits with Eddy's. Though he was a humorist, while she, as he satirized her, was humorless, they were both authors with public reputations to manage, images tied into their overall publicity strategy for advancing certain ideas in the marketplace.

The tableau of Twain's response as a reader and author to ideas in the chapter on the "Method of the Future" in *The Pen and The Book*, a book about publishing and publicizing books, captures the ethos of this volume. Mark Twain and Mary Baker Eddy were different in style, in profits, and in their approaches to publishing. In Twain's viewpoint, based on the marginalia he scribbled as he studied the matter, Eddy had mastered intuitively what Besant called "the Method of the Future," that is, the difference between the product and the selling of the product to the public, even if that product were a book, a personal reputation, or a spiritual or medical cure. Twain had scrawled in pencil above the chapter heading, "Nothing could be stupider than selling unrequired things by methods suitable to required—like salt, matches, tobacco." As Besant's chapter had explained, the method of the future was about publicity. The "performance" of the book occurred not in the writing, advertising, or selling in bookstores, but rather when the public bought it and talked about it, when the book entered the popular culture through the marketplace of ideas, taking on a life of its own, as it were. Marketing humorous books that were not "required," or selling religious books that were required of all believers, had to do with cultural storytelling, the process of branding, with creating a need that the product would fulfill. The same "method" shapes the advertising of disease today, as this book explains. Twain understood the method of the future to mean that authors, ministers, and doctors would all be in the same economic boat as Besant's chapter predicted, and as Twain agreed in his marginalia. Unless buyers thought a product was "required," it wouldn't sell, whether media, religion, or medicine.

The third chapter picks up the development of these ideas as they reoccur today, in the research of "regular" doctors, who are as individualistic and enterprising as any leader of any new religion in America has had to be. They have had to buck the prevailing attitudes of the status quo medical establishment in order to pursue their research about the role of faith in healing. The third chapter is intended as a representative reading of the research drawn from the National Library of Medicine at the National Institutes of Health, rather than a meta-analysis, for the body of literature is voluminous. The first research on prayer in healing was completed at the turn of the twentieth century, concurrently with the emergence of modern psychology, the Mind Cure, and New Thought movements. Between 1890 and 1970, there was more opportunity for research about prayer in foxholes than in clinical settings, and it wasn't until the rise of the American fascination with Eastern religions—with Transcendental Meditation, at the height of the drug culture of the 1960s and 1970s, and then with Buddhism from the 1980s until the present day—that doctors again took up the question. The third chapter highlights the controversies about clinical studies and therapeutic intervention through prayers and the ideas among leading physicians about the role of faith in healing.

In the fourth chapter, closely related to the research data on prayer, is the research about the brain, the stress-relaxation response and neuroimmunology, and the role of meditation in mind-body medicine. The work of leading neurologists is used to explain the stress-relaxation response, along with the role of popular medical advice books promoting this school of thinking about the relationship between emotions and biology in medicine. The substance of the biannual conferences of the Mind Life Institute, an organization of Buddhists and the neuroscientists involved in brain research involved in psychological and cognitive restructuring for heart patients, is discussed. So, too, is the news media's reaction when the Dalai Lama was invited to give the keynote speech to the annual convention of doctors of neuroscience. There were protests from all quarters about inviting a religious figure to speak to thousands of doctors and neuroscientists. The highly publicized negative reaction epitomizes the problem of the resistance to the ideas about the relationship between mental peace and wellness, and the role of the mass media in constructing that resistance by emphasizing negative publicity. Reactive press is balanced by the proactive part of the equation.

The fifth chapter explores how Big Pharma, through aggressive uses of proactive mass media, presents the strongest economic force possible in opposition to the ideas of alternative and complementary medicine, prayer, and meditation in therapeutic settings. The drug culture penetrates every American life without audiences being fully aware of the complex social forces responsible for the generation and consequences of this way of thinking. The intricacies of advertising science in popular media are explored: disease mongering through pharmaceutical corporations' unbranded disease awareness campaigns and through brand advertising. Key concepts from global health-care industries, and the communication and promotional strategies underlying the launch of new prescription drugs are described, drawing on a dozen current trade press books written by medical marketing experts. To understand fully the economic pressures about patented prescription drugs and the regulatory approval mechanism that either can slow or speed up the launch of new drugs into the global marketplace, a brief description of the economics of drug approval is provided. The bottom line is financial, and the numbers are in the billions. Other issues such as conflicts of interest among physicians, advertising in medical journals, the web of compromise in the funding of "nonprofit" consumer groups supported and in many cases established by pharmaceutical companies, and the role of lobbying in the drug culture infrastructure are raised as vital political issues that drive the economy.

I have tried diligently to present these arguments in a balanced and judicious manner, without bias or preferential treatment for any one school of thought or religious outlook. The interdependence of Eastern and Western ideas about religion and health informs the internal rationale for this book, and the intersection of American historical, literary culture with contemporary popular mediated culture constructs the infrastructure of this book.

My own religious perspectives are based in Catholicism, the religion into which I was baptized as a child and the religion of my ancestors and to which I belong. I am interested in Buddhism because of my reading over the past twenty years in the literature of the Christian mystics, and the writing of contemplative monks such as Thomas Merton. Among the Buddhist ideas that are particularly relevant to an ethic for the mass media, I subscribe to theories of dependent origination and the interdependence of all people; the importance of inner peace; and the role of suffering as a gateway to wisdom, to freedom from anxiety, and to the Middle Path that is through compassion, forgiveness, and healing silence through the Eastern and Western mental disciplines of contemplation.

My hope is that this book contributes to the growing body of knowledge in research and scholarship on media, religion, and culture. I do hope it is a tale well told, and has significance in positive and interesting, thought-provoking ways. May all who read these pages do so in good health!

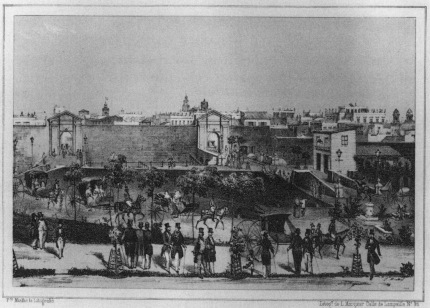

Figure 1.1: "Isla de Cuba. Puertas de Monserrate," by French artist
Federico Mialhe. Shows genteel women in carriages, men strolling
on the esplanade before the walls of Havana during the
height of the American "Invalid's Tour." Lithograph n. 96,
ca. 1830. Courtesy of the Cuban Heritage Collection.
University of Miami Libraries, Coral Gables, Florida.

Chapter 1

"MAN'S ACCIDENTS ARE GOD'S PURPOSES"
HARVARD AND HEROIC CURES

> We pass for what we are
> Character teaches above our wills.
> —Ralph Waldo Emerson, *Self-Reliance*

When the young wife of Nathaniel Hawthorne stood by her rain-streaked parlor window in the 1840s in Concord, Massachusetts, and used the stone in her wedding ring to etch into the glass the words "Man's Accidents are God's Purposes," she framed her own biographical narrative, one in which an invalid was rescued from death by a handsome, ruddy-cheeked novelist. Far from casting herself as the heroine in this romance, though, the narrative Sophia already had written as part of her daily female duty—for she was an intrepid journalizer in an age of diaries and letter-writing—was about a young lady's spiritual history through illness. Sophia belonged to the last generation of the women of preindustrial America who were not admitted to public schools, but who had access to the schools only in the evening or the summer, when the boys were resting or playing. Within that tradition, where girls were educated in front parlors, "reading" was commonly understood to mean elocution, "composition" was making copies, and "writing" was an exercise in journals and copy-books. An invalid much of her girlhood, she read philosophy, conversed with Rev. William Ellery Channing and Ralph Waldo Emerson, and painted Transcendental landscapes, full of skies with slanting rays from the sun shielded by luminous clouds, under the tutelage of the famous painters Washington Allston and Thomas Doughty. Her own spiritual history was a narrative typical in many ways of other women of her day, a story in which illness, religion, and romance were inextricably mixed.

Religion has influenced the directions and practice of American medicine since its earliest days, when the identity of the doctor and preacher were synonymous, as they were for Sophia Peabody. Historically, eminent physicians have seen themselves as healers. In this they were supported by patients who saw themselves as believers in a certainty that defined spiritual and medical authority, and their faith in that authority was unwavering, no matter how toxic the cure, nor how greatly they suffered from experimental prescriptions. Between the healer's role and the patient's was a Romantic attitude toward religion; without this, American medicine could not have advanced.[1]

MEDICO-SPIRITUAL AUTHORITY

Dr. Oliver Wendell Holmes declared the spirit of experiment and discovery that informed the field of medical science in the mid- to late nineteenth century when he welcomed the new class enrolled in Harvard Medical School in 1861. Holmes told the group of men assembled in the classroom "Science is the topography of ignorance," and "The best part of our knowledge is that which teaches us where knowledge leaves off and ignorance begins."[2] When Holmes had addressed a group of established doctors at the annual meeting of the Massachusetts Medical Society on May 30, 1860, about the "Currents and Cross-currents" in nineteenth-century medicine, he summarized another commonplace of the day, that "invalidism" was the "natural state" of many women: though it might degenerate into disease, it would never lead to full health, he concluded.[3] About the critical issues in the field of medicine, the eminent poet and physician declared, "There are many ladies . . . perpetually taking remedies for irremediable pains and back-aches and stomach-aches. . . . There is no doubt that the constant demand for medicinal remedies from patients of this class leads to their over-use."[4]

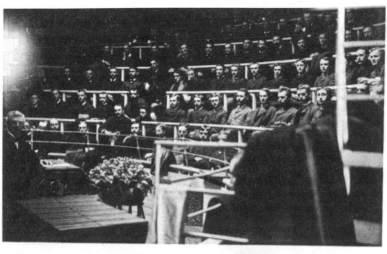

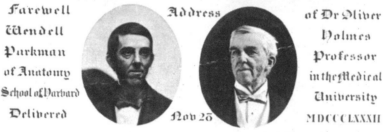

𝕱𝖆𝖗𝖊𝖜𝖊𝖑𝖑 𝕬𝖉𝖉𝖗𝖊𝖘𝖘 of 𝕯r 𝕺𝖑𝖎𝖛𝖊𝖗 𝖂𝖊𝖓𝖉𝖊𝖑𝖑 𝕳𝖔𝖑𝖒𝖊𝖘 𝕻𝖆𝖗𝖐𝖒𝖆𝖓 𝕻𝖗𝖔𝖋𝖊𝖘𝖘𝖔𝖗 of 𝕬𝖓𝖆𝖙𝖔𝖒𝖞 in 𝖙𝖍𝖊 𝕸𝖊𝖉𝖎𝖈𝖆𝖑 𝕾𝖈𝖍𝖔𝖔𝖑 𝖔𝖋 𝕳𝖆𝖗𝖛𝖆𝖗𝖉 𝖀𝖓𝖎𝖛𝖊𝖗𝖘𝖎𝖙𝖞 𝕯𝖊𝖑𝖎𝖛𝖊𝖗𝖊𝖉 𝕹𝖔𝖛 25 𝕸𝕯𝕮𝕮𝕮𝕷𝕏𝕏𝕏𝕀𝕀

1847   1882   Oliver Wendell Holmes

Figure 1.2: Oliver Wendell Holmes lecturing to the all-male class at Harvard Medical School, ephemera in commemoration of his farewell address. Holmes wrote, "science is the topography of ignorance." Farewell Address of Dr. Oliver Wendell Holmes: Parkman Professor of Anatomy in the Medical School of Harvard University. Photomechanical reproduction, ca. 1882. Courtesy of the National Library of Medicine.

From the standpoint of clinical trials, unregulated and lacking any scientific protocols, many experimental medicines were used on neurasthenic, genteel female patients of the nineteenth century, contributing to the development of medical knowledge. Given the extremes of these experiments, called "heroic cures," it is no wonder that so many people in the late nineteenth century gravitated toward alternatives to regular medicine, including herbs, exercise and diet, and water cures—the last they could read about in the *Water Cure Journal*. Archival research among the letters, journals, and diaries of the day constantly reiterates the finding of what seemed to be the expression of an age as anxious as our own. Every lady, it seemed, as well as some of the gentlemen, had some sort of "nervous" disorder, and physicians tried various prescriptions in an attempt to find a cure. Failing that, the individuals either died—or took a vacation journey and wrote about it, publishing a book or a family album of reminiscences.

Not unlike the welter of self-help and alternative medicine books found today in any franchised bookstore or busy metropolitan train station, books by physicians about popular maladies and how to cure them "naturally" were a staple of turn-of-the-century magazine, newspaper, and book publishing. Seldom were these writings grounded in science. They formed an amalgam of medical and spiritual advice, much of it couched in the domestic language of the day. In one slim volume, *Nervousness: A Brief and Popular Review of the Moral Treatment of Disordered Nerves*, a popular writer weighed in about the causes and cures of the ailment that made invalids of so many women. Dr. A. T. Schofield wrote, "England lagged behind America and France when it came to the treatment of nerves, hypochondria, hysteria and related maladies imaginaries. Primarily, the disease affected women from 'robust' families, whose daughters who (behind their backs) were said to be 'shamming.'"[5]

There was always an element of implied doubt about whether the illness was in the body or in the mind, which insinuated a further doubt about the moral character of the individuals in poor health. Had they done something to bring it on themselves? Were they just imagining the illness? Too much compassion shown to a young woman, some thought, was only said to be "encouraging her." So, perhaps, if a physician prescribed a rather painful cure as prescription, there might have been a greater willingness in the family to accept such a practice, thinking the individual might be shocked out of her complaints—brought to her senses, as it were. This type of neurasthenia, particularly among women, provided some physicians with the opportunity to link the "weaknesses" of the mind and the maladies of the body, to see the relationship between the sufferer's disposition and emotional outlook, connecting his or her conscious and unconscious intentions. Schofield wrote, "We may be said to live consciously and to exist unconsciously. The two powers are variously exercised; for while in health the conscious mind often acts to the detriment of the body, the unconscious never does, save when it is diseased."[6]

Of the types of mind sufferers, the medical literature distinguished two groups: the neurasthenic, who had weak nerves, and the neuromimetic, or hysteric who suffered from unconscious mind disorders.

> In nerve disease the mental sufferings are really mostly due to the fact that the conscious mind is, as a whole, sound, and hence can feel intensely the disordered state of the nervous system. This may show itself in dreads, fancies, fixed ideas, morbid thoughts, suspicions; or perhaps loss of memory of association, of vigor, of keenness of intellect, of quickness of feeling, of moral sense, or the faculties may be exaggerated in many ways. . . . The bodily sufferings may range from mere weakness to the agonies of almost every known disease, which can all be reproduced by the unconscious mind with perfect fidelity, even against the conscious will or wish of the person.[7]

Charles Darwin had similar symptoms and suffered from ill health all his life, fitting an "obvious pattern," according to one scholar, of "nervous dyspepsia." Nonetheless, he lived until age seventy-four, and his *Origin of the Species*, published in 1859, shaped the debates about science and religion in his age as well as our own, especially in contemporary debates about intelligent design and evolution. Yet he and the neurasthenic female shared what one author called the "Victorian Malady." Darwin apparently suffered from the ubiquitous headaches, "strong mental impressions," numbness, and a "peculiar uneasy feeling." Darwin's physicians believed in cold baths and toxic medicines. "Liquor potassae arsenitis, or Fowler's solution, and the mercury preparation, calomel, were considered to be useful in curing many disorders." Some physicians prescribed such toxins in a preventative mode; even after the attacks passed, the patient was supposed to continue to ingest the substance. The usual plan was to begin with small doses of the arsenic, and continue to increase it daily until the pain subsided: "Arsenic combined with calomel was useful as a purge. Neuralgia was treated with arsenic. . . . Problems resulting . . . from a morbid sensibility of the stomach and intestines" were treated with arsenic. Darwin's physician believed that side effects such as nausea, and tingling in the hands and feet "should not be viewed with alarm." Arsenic was good for everybody, well or ill, it was thought, for people who enjoyed very good health as a tonic, to give firmness and vigor to the constitution. Mercury and arsenic mixed was considered a good purgative. Physicians also believed that humidity, temperature of the atmosphere, and its "electricity" were beneficial.[8] In New England, as well as in London, many physicians who had used heroic doses of mercury and arsenic, usually to no avail, finally recommended what was commonly called the "invalid tour," a trip or vacation to a warmer climate, perhaps Italy or Cuba. From Boston, many shipped directly to Havana, a trip that Sophia Peabody made to escape the winter of 1833, staying until the spring of 1835.[9]

In the decade before she went to Cuba, Sophia Peabody lay ill with neurasthenic sufferings; there was not a great deal of respect for the reality of such nervous disorders, as Schofield observed, but there were continuing attempts to cure the lethargy with a variety of toxic cures. Only toward the last quarter of the nineteenth century, after the spreading popularity of mind cures, including mesmerism and all types of hypnotic quackery, did the medical establishment treat seriously the idea of hypochondria, or a diseased state of the imagination about the body and the mind.[10] Bad surroundings, association with other sufferers, worry, shock from bad news, and a lack of exercise were among the many known causes, "especially if dyspepsia be present." Symptoms were equally vague and amorphous, including headache, heart palpitations, sleeplessness, timidity or irritability, mental laziness, and apathy. In such cases, although drugs continued to be administered, often toxins in heroic doses, so many alternatives to regular medicine arose that finally doctors like Schofield concluded that "the therapeutic value of faith and hope, *though not in our textbooks*, is often enough to turn the scale in favor of recovery." Schofield concluded, "The power of mind over the body has limits, but they have never yet been ascertained. What a patient can do to cure himself, the forces he can set in action are as yet unknown. . . . Mental therapeutics may be directed by the patient himself to calming the mind in excitement, arousing feelings of joy, hope, faith, and love . . . by giving oneself the most favorable life suited to cure the disease."[11]

The belief that women and men alike invested in physicians was a type of religious faith. Similar to the social role of the preacher, the doctors' knowledge about medicine and religion was grounded in texts that were widely accepted as fact. Both the medical doctor and the preacher held a cultural authority grounded in public beliefs about narrative and literary truths, many of them romantic, defensible on the basis of "scientific" or biblical beliefs. In the mid- to late nineteenth century, when the ratio of clergy to physicians in the U.S. was roughly 1 clergyman for every 87 Americans, and 1 physician for every 618 Americans, in Massachusetts, there were about the same number of clergy as there were physicians on record (1,662 to 1,643), perhaps reflecting that the professions were often reported as being one and the same.[12]

NATURAL HEALING

The physician trained in medical schools such as Harvard tried to counteract nature. "Assaulting" illness, they prescribed not only mercury and arsenic but also alcohol, opium, and strychnine in order to "reinvigorate" the patients. For the founders of Harvard Medical School, men with the professional status and social standing of Oliver Wendell Holmes and Walter Channing, homeopathy, the science of "like cures like," was one of the many "sects loyal to cures" that characterized the scientific quarrels of the age, as medical historians have outlined.[13] (The histories of medicine, science, and society are academic disciplines in themselves. My purpose here is not to recapitulate the excellent research in these fields, but for purposes of my larger argument in this book, to highlight some of these sects and popular beliefs about healing, however briefly.) Begun in 1796, with the publication of the first scientific paper by the German physician Samuel Christian Hahnemann (1755–1843), homeopathy held that diseases were cured by agents capable or producing symptoms resembling those found in the disease under treatment.[14] When in 1842, the prominent Bostonian Holmes twice addressed the city's Society for the Diffusion of Useful Knowledge on the subject "Homeopathy and Its Kindred Delusions," he warned that the common ideas about homeopathy, such as one "might as well try it, " and "it can do no harm," actually would harm the medical establishment itself. He said, "It always does very great harm to the community to encourage ignorance, error, or deception in a profession which deals with . . . life and health. . . . So long as the body is affected through the mind, no audacious device, even of the most manifestly dishonest character . . . can fail of producing occasional good to those who yield it an implicit or even a partial faith."[15]

Holmes objected that

> [h]omeopathy has come before our public at a period when the growing spirit of eclecticism has prepared many ingenious and honest minds to listen to all new doctrines with a candor liable to degenerate into weakness . . . who have slid into the belief that matter subdivided becomes less material, and approaches nearer to a spiritual nature as it requires a more powerful microscope for detection. . . . Some persons seem disposed to take the ground . . . that the Laity must pass formal judgment between the Physician and the Homoeopathist, as it once did between Luther and the Romanists.[16]

Holmes observed that Hahnemann and his disciples constituted a "hostile" force against which physicians must speak out in "self-defence": "It began with an attempt to show the insignificance of all existing medical knowledge." The homoeopathists invented a name, Holmes charged, for all those who were trained in formal medicine, from Hippocrates to Hunter, calling them all "allopathists," and by doing so drew the "line," "lifted the lance," "sounded the charge, and are responsible for any little skirmishing which may happen."[17]

As Holmes continued to lecture, he outlined the physician's knowledge about anatomy, physiology, and chemistry, all advancing areas of science and part of the curriculum at Harvard Medical School.

The "borderline" to which Holmes alluded distinguished plants from metals in pharmacology. He urged medical students not to be "childish" in their "condemnation" of a particular class of agents in medicine, Holmes said, specifically mercury and arsenic. Though "disturbing" to the system, Holmes lectured, mercury's efficacy in certain forms of disease is acknowledged by all but the most sceptical [sic] theorists . . . calling it a "great panacea" for women's pelvic diseases, though he warned that there were many abuses of the mineral, and should not be used for all ailments.[18] Similarly, "arsenic-eating may improve the conditions of both horses and of human beings for a time," he argued, as could copper and other metal "intrusive" into the animal organization of the body. "The constitution bears slow poisoning a great deal better than might be expected," but members of the medical establishment were getting out of the habit of prescriptions so strong that they produced death and caused malpractice lawsuits. "Medical experience is a great thing, but we must not forget that there is a higher experience, which tries its results in a court of a still larger jurisdiction; that, namely in which the laws of human belief are summoned to the witness-box, and obliges to testify to the sources of error which beset the medical practitioner." Holmes concluded his opening lecture by saying the "the bedside is always the true center of medical teaching."[19]

DR. WALTER CHANNING

Certainly the thinking about healing and medicine that characterized the Harvard Medical School establishment opinion in the lectures of Dr. Oliver Wendell Holmes was consistent with that of his colleague, Dr. Walter Channing (1786–1876), Dean of the Faculty of Harvard Medical School from 1829 to 1847, a founding editor of the *New England Journal of Medicine* in the 1820s, professor of Midwifery and Medical Jurisprudence at Harvard, and Sophia Peabody's personal physician. Channing claimed the "discovery" of using ether for childbirth and in other medical procedures for Boston, and for Harvard, though actually it had been used elsewhere earlier. Few could read about Channing's life, or see the dignity in his lined face in the oil portrait hanging in the library at Harvard Medical School, without seeing in his biography both the tragic and the heroic, the realism of his character amidst personal failure and professional triumph that marked many lives as heroic, in the sense that the twentieth-century American novelist William Faulkner later claimed for all human life: endurance against all odds. For despite Channing's sincerest, best efforts to alleviate pain in childbirth, many women died. To read about the standards of obstetrics in this period, when puerperal fever could have been averted by the simple act of a physician washing his hands after examining a cadaver, is to understand the fear that must have informed every young married woman's life. Death and the horrors of childbirth would have forced even the most disbelieving into a state of prayerful supplication to a spiritual authority they imagined as male and merciful.

To Channing's great anguish, he attempted to deliver his second wife, Eliza, of a stillborn son after she had endured fourteen hours of labor, a son she conceived at forty years of age well into three years of marriage. Dr. Channing concluded that "the baby could not be born by natural means and that instruments must be used," according to his biographer.[20] Though "wiser heads should have counseled him against it," Channing himself performed the necessary operation on his wife, who died a half hour later from hemorrhaging. "Channing fell apart," according to Harvard medical historian Amelie Kass, after watching his wife bleed to death. The tragedy was but one of a series of unexpected deaths among his circle at a time when cholera also infected the city.[21]

Channing is an intriguing figure precisely because he was among those leaders in the emerging medical profession whose prescriptions caused serious, sometimes lethal side effects, and yet he was respected and believed. People understood his own frailty, and no doubt he was a man of conscience and in his anguish felt his culpability. The death of his second wife must have made it difficult to raise his remaining children: his son Ellery, named after Walter's brother, Rev. Ellery Channing, the famous preacher, turned out to be a weak and troubled man who married the younger sister of Margaret Fuller, the great champion of education and women's rights and author of *Women in the Nineteenth Century*. She of course later chose to die in a shipwreck with her Italian husband, whom she had met during her travels to Italy, a man some years her junior who reportedly did not speak much English. There was an acceptance of death among Bostonians in the nineteenth century that we have to strive to understand, so great has been the progress in medicine. Death was, to say the least, a commonplace. The only experience we have in the twenty-first century is the experience of being part of a televisual audience witnessing the causalities of war in the Middle East, or famine in Africa, or casualties from natural disasters. After awhile, it must be said, a certain insensitivity to the suffering of others sets in, as the numbing effect of the reality of death and suffering drives the electronic audience inward spiritually, exacerbating the anxieties associated with the psychology of the self and its many maladies, both real and imagined.

It was, after all, not the quaint home remedy grown in the garden and administered at the hearth but the heroic cure and the toxins used to heal that could also kill that informed the thinking about medicine responsible for shaping the future of medical education in America.

According to textbooks of the day, the medical education curriculum at the time consisted of anatomy, pathology, *materia medica* and/or pharmacy, chemistry, surgery, and midwifery or the diseases of women and children. In some schools, medical students received training in medical jurisprudence, or training in the art of defending oneself in a court of law. The latter became one of Channing's areas of expertise. Though the field of medical law was just emerging, by the end of the century, the attempts by Christian Scientists to practice not medicine "but a type of hopefulness" would constitute a significant influence on the shape of the body of malpractice laws.[22]

Praising a new book in a review for a medical journal, Channing commented on the utility of a text written by a physician who had practiced for seventeen years before going into law. The book, titled *A Medico-Legal Treatise on Malpractice and Medical Evidence, comprising the Elements of Medical Jurisprudence*, was written by John Elwell, M.D., member of the Cleveland Bar.[23] It covered ideas only barely introduced into medical education, including malpractice, evidence, moral (as opposed to intellectual) insanity, poisons, infanticide, wounds, rape, inquests, and "criminal abortion," which was "widespread" in Massachusetts and Boston in 1860. Ewell acknowledged the legal problem with using poisons for abortions: they sometimes produced lifelong invalidism. "We have no specifics for producing abortion," Channing wrote, and even where women brought the abortion on themselves, he did not think physicians should avoid such patients for fear of malpractice suits. Such cases were difficult to prosecute where criminal doctors practiced illegally, Channing wrote, because women usually went to the doctors unaccompanied. In one instance he cited, the woman went with a friend, and though she died of the abortion, the doctor married the friend, the only witness, and though the doctor was suspected of the crime and arrested, little could be done to prosecute him.[24] He concluded that the law was often useless in these cases of medical malpractice. Yet the medical education of a physician ought to include training in how to behave in court, Channing argued, because at some point the doctor might be called into court as a defendant, witness, or plaintiff. Channing argued that, when summoned, the physician should not resist because that could lead to charges of contempt, leading to a fine or imprisonment.

Channing's other teaching specialty was the development of the profession of obstetrics, or midwifery, a field the doctors fiercely protected from women practitioners, even as morbidity rates were lower among midwives than among doctors because they did not conduct autopsies and spread puerperal fever through contact with cadavers.[25] The practice of etherization in childbirth, for example, was "invented" at Harvard, as Channing claimed in his book on the subject published more than a decade after his wife died. In the fall of 1846, Channing wrote in his 400-page book published by Ticknor & Fields, *A Treatise on Etherization in Childbirth Illustrated by Five-Hundred and Eighty-One Cases*, published in 1848. Channing at first had published his own pamphlets, then he collected the experiences of other physicians in the Boston area, who contributed letters, opinions, and cases, publishing the results in the book's compilation. His sole object in developing this remedy to pain, according to his treatise, was to determine if the use of chloroform and ether was safe for the mother and child.[26] Though there were dangers if the sponge was unclean or if too much ether were administered, reaching the brain and causing death, Channing believed in the practice wholeheartedly. "Etherization in midwifery has been employed here now for a year," he wrote, "and, with some industry, my collections of cases do not much exceed five hundred. I have no doubt that many more exist; but of the certain, I know of those only of which I give reports. The number is not large. But just add them to the hundreds and thousands which are furnished from abroad."[27] All told and accounted for, Channing concluded, they showed the practice to be safe.

The ether rendered the woman physically limp and powerless to participate in the birth process, of course, and put her labor entirely into the hands of the attending physician. Channing's lengthy treatise describes the state of "perfect repose" among women after the administration of ether in labor, and breathing that is "perfectly noiseless." He summarized the prevailing belief that the pain of childbirth resulted not from the contractions themselves, but from the "resistance to the contractions of the womb, which the moving body, the foetus, encounters in its progress to birth . . . by taking away the disturbing actions of the will," relief from unnecessary pain occurred.[28]

Religious objections to etherization grounded in scripture "reached the pulpit," according to Channing. The argument against ether used

Genesis 3:16, "Unto the woman he said . . . In sorrow thou shalt bring forth children." One physician objected to Channing's use of ether, writing that "the very suffering which a woman undergoes in labor is one of the strongest elements in the love she bears her offspring. I have fears for the moral effect of this discovery, both on the patient and on the physician."[29]

Channing also consulted his Bible, ruminating. He concluded that the meaning of that passage might mean that the sorrow a woman experiences would be from the conduct of her children. Perhaps he also was referring inadvertently to the conduct of his own children. He defended the use of chloroform and ether because they "resulted from natural intelligence and natural laws." Channing remained uncertain about the "precise meaning" of the sentence in Genesis referred to, and "doubtful whether it meant DOOM or PROPHECY" and so he referred the debate to theologians. A public debate ensued, including publication of pamphlets by clergy on both sides of the question. Channing wrote, "The interest of our subject has extended beyond the medical profession, and has even reached the pulpit. One sermon used as its text 'Deliver us from evil.' And it 'excited some interests.' When a woman was asked, upon leaving the church, how she liked the sermon against etherization, she said, 'Very Well. It is not wholly wrong to lessen or destroy pain. WE MAY EAT PEPPERMINTS!'"[30]

The moral objection argued that ether was like morphia, opium, and laudanum, and might be inhaled "for the intellectual excitement it produces, and is used for pleasure." Channing argued fiercely against the idea that ether was used for pleasure. He defended his employment of the drug for medicinal use, to alleviate pain, especially women's pain in childbirth that so often ended in death.[31]

In the years following 1840, heroic medicine fell from popular favor in America, according to the medical historian Fuller, in part because Parisian medical schools constituted a competitive force. They had trained their doctors to diagnose illness rather than attack it; they studied anatomy, and even used stethoscopes.[32] Other popular cures, including homeopathy, hydropathy, and mind cures, rapidly took the place of belief and trust in traditional heroic and experimental medicine.

In 1844, twenty-eight years after the "invention" of the stethoscope, homeopathic doctors formed the first national medical organization, the

American Institute of Homeopathy. With the founding of the American Medical Association in 1847, "regular" doctors differentiated themselves as a profession from homeopaths, and in this they were supported whole-heartedly by the American newspapers.[33] In 1880, Walter Channing and a group of other doctors organized a society for those practicing in psychiatry and neurology, and over the following twenty-five years devoted themselves to working with the state to develop hospitals and favorable legislation for the care of the "insane." For the first five years of the existence of this new organization, Walter Channing served as its secretary, and as its first president in 1892. Regarding the future of medicine, he forcast: "it is impossible to explain mental disease-forms and mental symptoms in terms of structure because we have no knowl-edge of the relation between normal mental functions and the anatomi-cal arrangements of the brain. . . . I believe we shall become one united branch of medicine."[34]

The American Medical Association and traditionally educated doc-tors also strove to separate their profession from ministers who prayed with patients, or worse yet, those who dispensed spiritual advice along with natural remedies. The established physicians, whose practices sometimes did result in the death of patients, had to be concerned with jurisprudence and malpractice, at the same time, as they were working to elevate as well as "secure their social and economic status."[35] Among the American Medical Association's earliest resolutions was an attempt to associate homeopathy with non-American medicine and "foreigners," and to distance themselves from "volunteer missionaries" or clergy who gave homeopathic advice.[36] If, as many historians have stated, a "wall" developed between religion and medicine in the twentieth century, it arose because the profession of the physician needed to distance itself from spiritualists, in order to establish the credibility so vital to the belief processes that inform the patient-provider communication and lead to effective treatment, to healing, and to cures.

The American medical establishment represented by the founders of Harvard Medical School, and the generation of Drs. Walter Channing and Oliver Wendell Holmes, changed in response not only to competi-tive pressures from medical education abroad, but to the pressures for alternatives to standard medical practices from the press and from a changing popular culture. Historians have noted that just as science became more secularized, "metaphysical causality" infused many of the less scientific, unorthodox approaches to medicine.[37] Popular beliefs about health and well-being tended to favor medicines grown in the garden, and magical cures such as mesmerism.[38]

THE MEDICAL ADVICE BOOK

The ideas about botanical cures were popularized by Samuel Thompson (1769–1843) in his 1822 edition of the *Botanic Family Physician*. Advertising its aim, "to make every man his physician," the book sold thousands of copies, resulting in the formation of healing societies and journals. Because Thompson had whetted the appetites of the public for new ideas about home cures, they were ripe for homeopathy, hydropathy, and electricity as popular approaches to medicine over the subsequent decades. As medical historians have described, hydropathy was as popular as homeopathy. Its historical roots date to as early as 1723, with the publication of an American edition of John Smith's book, *Curiosities of Common Water*, in Philadelphia. Dr. Joel Shew of New York developed the idea of water as a brand: water was given orally, and as a healing agent externally.[39]

The popular homeopathy of Hahnemann's work, *Organon of the Rational Art of Healing* (1810), strove to offer not only a consistency between symptoms and prescriptions, but also a unique method of lowering dosages and administering only one drug at a time, instead of mixing high doses of several drugs, so that the effect of each was indistinguishable. Hahnemann's "infinitesimals" theory central to homeopathy resulted in highly diluted doses. The tremendous popularity of homeopathy motivated "ordinary" allopathic physicians to organize professionally against the encroachment of self-help medicine, and to form the American Medical Association, according to historians.[40]

Haller wrote that homeopathy owed its popularity to the skepticism among physicians about long-standing procedures such as bleeding, cupping, heroic dosages, and other brutal cures. Hahnemann concluded after much study that "the curative basis of medicines in the *materia medica* stemmed from their power to induce in healthy persons symptoms analogous to the diseases for which they were administered."

"What incurred the wrath of the regulars, according to Haller," was not so much Hahnemann's first principle as the heretical assertions that quickly followed, including his belief that diseases resulted from neither mechanical nor chemical changes of the body but from spiritual, dynamic disturbances of life." He supported mesmerism, where the physician put his hand over affected parts. "Until Hahnemann moved in the direction of infinitesimal doses, much of his theory brought praise."[41]

The fourth American edition of the homeopathic classic, *The Manual of Homeopathic Practice and Symptomology* (1861), by C. H. G. Jahr, was published in New York by William Radde, the "sole agent" for the Leipzig Central Homeopathic pharmacy. Radde also served as an apothecary, advertising that "he has always on hand a good assortment of the best homeopathic medicines." Precise information about dosages and manners of application make up the twelve-hundred-page, one-volume textbook, preceded by a Table of Medicines (table of contents), which included prescriptions such as the following: vinegar, black snake root, hog's lard, wine, onion, garlic, aloe, clay, ambergris, ammonia, coal, poison of the honey-bee, arsenic, asparagus, mountain parsley, gold, camphor, mercury, hemp, lime, cayenne pepper, castor, horseradish, cucumber, saffron, rattlesnake poison, fox-glove, iron, strawberry, gentian, indigo, potash, magnesia, quicksilver, nickel, nitric-acid, acetate of morphia, pine, lead, poison oak, tomato, tin, thorn-apple, stronian, sulphuric acid, tobacco, turpentine, stinging nettle, and witch hazel.[42]

Hydropathy, or water cures using baths and wet sheets offering "noninvasive, hygienic," and natural materials instead of drugs, resulted in the popular publications, *The Water-Cure Manual*, a periodical, and *The Hydropathic Encyclopedia*; a college; and a number of mineral baths and springs.[43] In America, hydropathy was popularized by many. Hydropathy was consistent with vegetarianism, and thought to be curative for illnesses of the nerves and digestive tract—perfect for the neurasthenic female whose ailments were so difficult to diagnose.[44]

Sylvester Graham (1794–1851) a Presbyterian minister by training, became "a temperance lecturer in 1830," according to historians. He preached not only moderation in consumption of alcohol, but also in dress and in food. His ideas melded the ideas of moderation, cleanliness, and godliness, all of that leading to salvation. According to historians,

he held lectures, "at some of which he had more than two thousand people," and publicized his ideas through books, pamphlets, health papers,
Ladies' Physiological Reform Societies, and Men's Graham boarding
houses. In 1838, the Grahamite American Health Convention in Boston
resolved to spread the gospel, and in 1839, his lectures and testimonials
about the health effects of regular bathing and whole wheat bread were
published, titled *Lectures on the Science of Human Health*.[45] Among those he
convinced were the Concord transcendentalists, and the utopian community, led by A. Bronson Alcott. Ellen White, foundress of the "second
largest religious denomination to emerge in the United States," according to Fuller, also subscribed to Graham's ideas and incorporated dietary
laws into the practices of the Seventh-Day Adventists. Through White's
popularization of the health food industry, she attracted the attention of
John Harvey Kellogg and C. W. Post.[46]

The popular culture "confused" ideas inherent in phrenology, mesmerism, animal magnetism, faith healing, and "the galvanism of Mr.
Samuel F. B. Morse," according to historians. "Western newspapers in
the 1840s were filled with strange goings-on. 'Professors' made the legs
of dead frogs jump, communicated with persons in adjoining rooms,
'read minds,' and put people into trances in which they sometimes
remembered seeing things which they had never seen before."[47]

The need to believe that cures were possible, outside of heroic medicine, and the popularization through the press of alternative medicine
converged with the Zeitgeist of the age—an interest in the power of
the mind, in psychology, and in the religious imagination. Dr. Phineas
Parkhurst Quimby, who was not trained as anything but a watch-
maker, saw a mesmerist by coincidence one day. From there, he began a
practice in New England that used a trance: according to historians, he
had many imitators in the medicine shows of the West.[48] Quimby liked
the idea of the higher power, as had many a utopian dreamer liked farm-
ing, without having to deal with the reality of weeds or dirt. Quimby
coined the term, adapted from the popular culture, that disease was an
imaginary thing, not real, and could be ameliorated not by a healer, like
a physician, but by a medium—a job for a man like himself. If one would
just "think himself in perfect health," he would find himself so. One
might say this current in American medical-religious thought resulted in

the positivist school of Norman Vincent Peale, Robert Schuller's many books and Crystal Cathedral, and more recently, Rick Warren's *Purpose-Driven Life*. The idea is that if one's head is screwed on straight, and one thinks positively about higher powers (not necessarily the equivalent of the Divine or God), then a person's good fortunes would fall into place, especially with regard to the body. This thinking is in the same vein as those who explained invalidism in the 1820s as being something that resulted from a defect in one's moral character.

This approach raises, in addition, the specter of blame in illness and misfortune. Self-reliance, or seeing the physical as the interlocutor between a spirit, psyche, and physical world, no doubt offered comfort to many uneducated people who had experienced the rigors of heroic medicine. In the positivist thinking of Quimby, a utilitarian view of mental power based on an economy of ideas was one more idea among many in an era well known and described by historians as filled with "quacks and eclectics in the borderline field between medicine and psychology."[49]

QUACKERY

The marginal idea of the parts of the mind controlling parts of the body was at once taken seriously and laughable, in the sense of what popular culture made of them in the pseudoscience of phrenology. Quimby, for example, had manipulated the scalp, passed his hands over the head, so that the electrical charge from his hands would activate certain organs. Joseph Rodes Buchanen graduated from the University of Louisville in medicine in 1842, and between 1846 and 1856 he led the Cincinnati Eclectic Institute, publishing a pamphlet the year he graduated from medical school outlining his ideas about phrenology; he went on to categorize ninety-one different functions of the brain.[50]

Two hundred years ago there was a robust marketplace for ideas that represented alternatives to regular medicine, some of it quackery and some of it on the side of the natural healing offered by botanicals and home remedies, or "domestic medicine" in which self-care and religion were mixed. Books such as the leatherbound, 730-page *Medical Companion or Family Physician*, by James Ewell, dedicated to Thomas Jefferson, was so popular that it went through eight editions in twelve years. It included a table of medicines for family use, with doses and quantities;

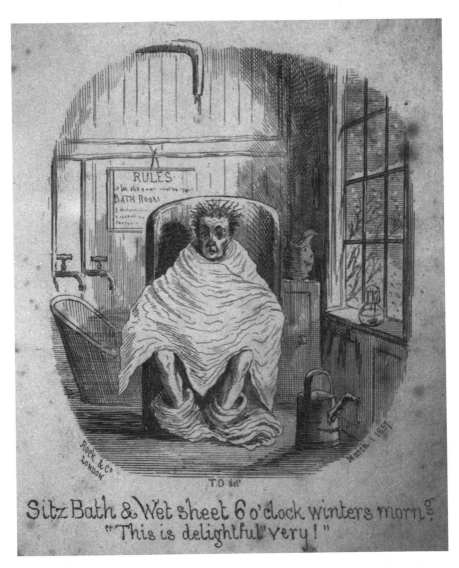

Figure 1.3: Cartoon of the "dawn sitz bath," a universally popular
water cure of the mid-nineteenth century. Sitz bath & wet sheet:
6 o'clock winters morning. Illustrated by Onwhyn Thomas in
Pleasures of the Water Cure (London: Rock & Co). Lithograph,
ca. 1857. Courtesy of the National Library of Medicine.

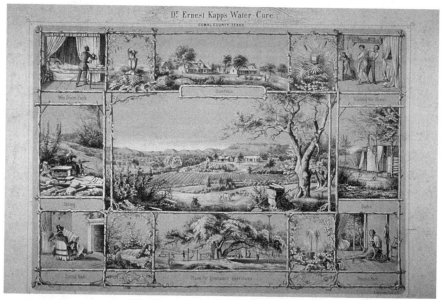

Figure 1.4: Dr. Ernest Knapp's water cure. *Comal County, Texas.*
Illustrated by G. Kraetzer. Lithograph, ca. 1850s.
Courtesy of National Library of Medicine.

a collection of recipes of compound medicines; and stated in its preface
that it was written specifically for Americans, by an American, ready
to treat "almost every disease to which the human body is subject, to
give their common names and surest symptoms, to point out the causes
whence they originate, treatment and prevention." Ewell's advertisement
included a list of natural herbs and plants in a *materia medica*, "pointing
out those precious samples wherewith God has graciously stored our
meadows, fields, and woods, for the healing of our diseases, and render-
ing us happily independent of foreign medicines, which, while they are
sometimes hard to be obtained, are frequently adulterated and always
costly."[51] Integrating poetry, the author's lengthy chapter on "the art of
preserving health" included food, exercise, sleep, love, hope, joy, fear,
anger, hatred, envy, avarice, temperance, vanity, dress, and religion.[52]

Acknowledging that the reader in 1820 or 1834 might have been
surprised to encounter the subject of religion in a guide to maintaining
health, the author warned against extremes of every kind in religion,
including superstition and enthusiasm. These pitfalls were illustrated by a

lengthy anecdote about a young woman whose once cheerful countenance was undermined by anxiety and melancholy, and soon "the fiends were waiting to receive her soul, and plunge it into the bitter torments of hell." Once her mind was calmed, her nerves restored, "I successfully counteracted the baleful effects of Superstition by the wholesome infusion of real Religion, and restored her to health," Ewell wrote.[53] He also stated:

> It is that fervent love of God and man, constituting the heart-gladdening religion of Christ, which I mean. This teaches us to deny ourselves, and follow in the exercise of all virtues, wherein consists the life or religion, laying aside all idle quarrels, self-interest, and needless debates about circumstantials; for this religion is not in words, but in works. . . . The man who loves God, enjoys . . . the consciousness of having placed his affections on the only object that truly deserves them. O! how amiable is gratitude; especially when directed to the Supreme Benfactor. . . . Cheerfulness is consistent with every species of virtue and practice of religion. It bears the same friendly regard to the mind as to the body; it banishes all anxious care and discontent, sooths and composes the passions, and keeps the soul in a perpetual calm. . . . My name is Religion. I am the offspring of Truth and Love, and the parent of Benevolence, Hope and Joy. That monster from whose power I have freed you, is called Superstition; she is the child of Discontent, and her followers are Fear and Sorrow.[54]

Ewell the physician turned to preaching, emphasizing the importance of maintaining a daily ritual or practice that integrated reflection into a regime, citing a fellow physician who had lived a long and healthy life:

> Throughout his whole life, as soon as he arose in the morning, which was generally very early, to retire for an hour to private prayer and meditation on some part of the Scriptures. He often told his friends, when they asked him how it was possible for him to go through so much fatigue, that it was this which gave him spirit and vigour in the business of the day. . . . For nothing, he said, could tend more to the health of the body, than the tranquility of the mind; and that he knew nothing which could support himself or his fellow-creatures, amidst the various distresses of life, but a well grounded confidence in the Supreme Being, upon the principles of Christianity.[55]

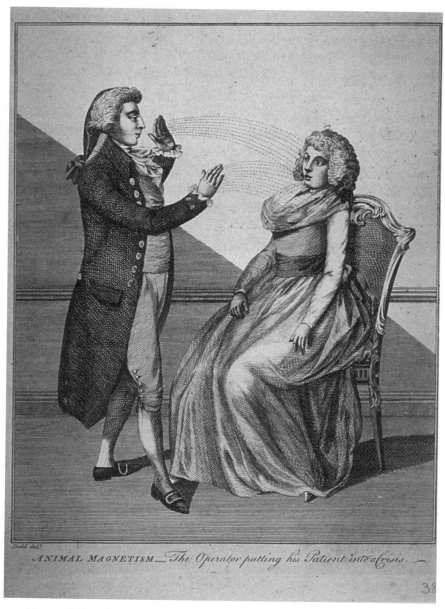

ANIMAL MAGNETISM—*The Operator putting his Patient into a Crisis.*

Figure 1.5: *The male hypnotist attempting to put a woman into a trance. Animal Magnetism: The Operator putting his Patient into a Crisis. Illustrated by Dodd. Engraving, London, 1794. Courtesy of the National Library of Medicine.*

Today, the issue of guilt and blame in medicine, and the industry in popular books about self-help and self-care that equate virtuous living with good health, is as robust as it was when Ewell argued that "it is in an ill man's interest there should be no God, because then there should be no punishment for sin, and though this interest passes into argument, yet it is never so conclusive as to pass into an entire satisfaction; for we cannot believe any person that has the use of his rational faculties, and gives himself the liberty of thinking, can deny the existence of a Deity, both as to creation and providence."[56]

Ewell's one-hundred-page compendium of vegetable-and-plant based cures and their applications also began with a mix of biblical and patriotic religion:

> How wonderful are thy works, O Lord! in wisdom hast thou made them all: the earth is full of riches! . . . In no department . . . do mingled wisdom and goodness shine with greater luster than in the animal kingdom. . . . The American continent, though the last found, is not the least favored of God in this respect. . . . The common saying, that every country contains the best cures for its own diseases, seems fully verified in America.[57]

This, then, was a popular phenomenon, clearly fueled by the public reaction to the image of and collective memory of failures of regular medicine in America. Along with the rich tradition of home remedies, plant-based cures mixed with religion in popular books on the library shelf by hearth and home, just as the medical establishment became professionalized. In 1851, apothecaries, or druggists, formed themselves into the American Pharmaceutical Association. In 1872, the doctors set up a committee specifically to communicate with the pharmacists, and by 1876 accepted recommendations on dosages and effects from the specialists educated in drugs.[58]

In 1879, the American Medical Association ruled that the advertising of drugs in medical journals was unethical; in 1884, the organization denounced doctors who endorsed drugs; and in 1888, the American Medical Association passed a formal motion to "disapprove" of any clergy or religious press "who recommended charlatans."[59] "By 1891, there were close to 14,000 homeopaths in the U.S. and more than 80,000 regular doctors," and by 1902, the physicians' association created a committee on medical education to evaluate the 155 medical schools in the country, a move that led to licensing. In 1897, the osteopaths, who used applications of heat and cold without drugs, founded the American Osteopathic Association, but chiropractors were less organized as a profession. In 1906, the fifty-ninth U.S. Congress passed the pure food and drug bill that required printing "approved by the Pure Food and Drug Act of 1906" on labels and on advertising.[60]

HEROIC PATIENTS

For people living in Boston or London during the first three decades of the nineteenth century and who suffered an ailment as minor as a persistent headache, mercury would have been prescribed—and in heavy doses. For trained medical doctors, mercury was among the most widely used and popularly administered substances in the early nineteenth century, especially when the doctor could think of nothing better to prescribe or had no idea about the diagnosis. According to one physician writing in the preface to his first American edition guiding the use of its application, "Instead of being prescribed to fulfill clear and well defined indications, such as blood-letting, opium, and most other efficient remedies, is not mercury by many rather given as a specific, or for symptoms of disease for which they know not what to give. It is acknowledged, that the difficulties connected with this subject are more easily pointed out than corrected."[61] Mercury is still used in vaccinations today, as the last chapter of this book addresses, and is thought by some to be responsible for the widespread epidemic of autism in children. Some were concerned enough about mercury used in dental fillings that a type of hysteria induced by widespread press coverage occurred during the 1990s, and people went to dentists to have all their dental work redone. No similar hysteria has occurred about the use of mercury and its connection with autism, which is underreported by the mainstream press.

Introduced into New England to fight inflammatory fevers early in American medical history, mercury quickly became a "fashionable remedy," thought by many physicians to be "indispensable," and fraught with controversy "with regard to its modus operandi," few could agree on the "time, manner, and degree of its use." According to A. W. Ives,

M.D., writing in an appendix to a book about the use and application of arsenic and mercury for heroic cures,

> Each one has marked out imaginary rules for the regulation of his own practice: and though he may perhaps find himself unable to explain definitely . . . the reasons on which his judgment is determined, or the precise object which he designs to fulfill, still he thinks, there are certain symptoms, which he has learned from observation to regard as indicating a condition of the system which calls for the medicinal influence of a mercurial course. Indeed so imperfect and unsettled is our knowledge on this subject, that no one can be impugned for empiricism, how improper soever his practice may appear; for there is no inconsistency so extravagant that it cannot be supported by precedent, and no hypothesis so absurd, that is cannot be defended by books.[62]

According to Kass's excellent biography of Dr. Walter Channing, Sophia Peabody was "one of his most interesting patients."[63] Sophia was a teenager when Channing took on her case, visiting her in her bedchamber regularly, according to her own description in her diaries and journals of the 1825–1833 period.[64] According to Kass's interpretation, Sophia "had suffered migrane headaches and other assorted ailments for several years and spent most of her time confined to her bedchamber. Channing . . . gently coaxed her out of the lethargy that had become a part of her existence." Though Kass is accurate in her interpretation that Sophia continued to admire Channing, Kass is incorrect about Sophia's "lethargy," the common cultural assumption about invalid women during the nineteenth century. One might rethink this conclusion, and suggest that what amounted to a period of internment in her bedroom—where she read at least a book a day when able and painted large, if ill-designed transcendentalist landscapes—was a reaction to the heroic prescriptions of arsenic and mercury, rather than to any defect of character. As an examination of her *Cuba Journals* demonstrates, when she escaped the prescriptions of her physician, she regained her health, though the experience of being an invalid never left her self-perception and larger moral sense of submission to "God's purposes."

Near death in 1829 from mercury and arsenic prescribed by Channing, Sophia was instructed by transcendentalist preachers of the period.

Among them, Rev. William Ellery Channing stood at her bedside and preached a sermon titled, "The Adaptation of Our Condition to Our Peculiar Wants," as she lay gravely ill from the mercury and arsenic.[65]

So while mercury along with other toxins was widely prescribed by physicians, in New England and in London during the mid-nineteenth century, mercury was often given to counteract the lethargy that was among the side effects of heroic cures. Used among female patients, it was thought to stimulate the action of the heart and arteries. Used as commonly as aspirin is today, and often prescribed not only in large doses, it was mixed with other toxins such as calomel. In a study of Charles Darwin, one scholar described his maladies as similar to those described by the typical neurasthenic female: he also was prescribed arsenic.[66]

In the midst of her distress, Sophia Peabody developed a theology of suffering, accepting her dosage as part of God's will for her. She described how it felt to ingest the mercury and arsenic in her diary: "There is continuously a black, iron hand pressed upon my brow, and the more buoyantly I spring forward to hear the music & gaze at the fountains, so much the more deeply do the iron fingers press. . . . It has extravagant transport & makes me listen to GOD in the still voice—it says, 'Were thy pathways here all roses, where would be the victory—where would be the need of a better land. GOD is in the lightening [sic] & the tempest & the whirlwind—in this iron hand.'"[67] It is difficult to discern whether the stimulant effects came from the drugs or from the preaching about her illness that also surrounded her.

She described in her journals how it felt to be on mercury and arsenic:

> To night I felt like the embodied spirit of pain. What are these agonizing twinges coming to? It seems as if my veins were finer than a cambric needle and that through them a deluge of fiery metal was struggling to wend, all but bursting the narrow pass. And what a singular elation of mind it brings with it. I could study Hebrew or hieroglyphics or solve to abstrusest problems better now than ever if my eyes would keep steady and could see. Am I and my body one? What a mystery! With all this pain pressing on me would I go hence? . . . Darkness hangs over the future. I am not near enough to the throne to tire of the scenes and joys of the world! Then I have not been long enough in it. There is dust on my spirit. The breath of holiness has not been strong

enough to disperse It. I do believe that Sickness and Pain and some of the highest ministers of God's inexpressible love.[68]

Yet some did call mercury and arsenic in heroic dosages quackery, even in Boston. One Boston physician objected in a pamphlet titled "Quackery Exposed!!!" He asked,

> Can it be made to appear reasonable, to any man in his sober senses, that the same medicine which will destroy the health, and perhaps the life of a well man, will in the hands of a skilful Physician cure a sick one? Away with such nonsense. Let reason and common sense be our guides; strip the profession of medicine of everything that looks like mystery, let the Physicians write their prescriptions in plain and intelligible language, that can be understood by the common people, and there would soon be a tremendous reaction in the public mind. . . . [This] would be preferred to the deadly effects of those poisonous minerals, mercury, arsenic &c. with which the shops of the apothecary and druggist are crammed.[69]

As much as Dr. Walter Channing was a model physician, a dedicated professional in the emerging field of medical education, along with other men struggling to learn how to be healers, he helped make Harvard a brand name in medicine synonymous with authority, intelligence, and compassion for the suffering. Yet it was women like Sophia Peabody, the prototypical neurasthenic female, whose passivity made possible the medical, cultural, and literary authority enjoyed by doctors, and whose religious endurance of heroic cures advanced American medicine. Many women like Sophia were models of submissiveness to claims of medical, religious, and literary importance; they had little recourse but to flee physically from the potency of mixing medical prescriptions and religion. Dr. Channing was only one of the several physicians who attended her, prescribing various cures, so when he prescribed the trip to Cuba, she must have been eager to leave the confinement of her bedroom and get on shipboard.[70]

The relationship between Sophia Peabody and her physician Dr. Walter Channing was a friendly and personal one, especially between the years 1828 and 1833, when she took the arsenic and mercury and was ill. In August 14, 1828, Channing wrote to her, prescribing in a jaunty tone "my latest prescription." His letter expressed a tolerance for the experimental nature of his prescriptions, as did her tone in her diaries express a resignation to her role as the subordinate in the relationship. Channing's prescription was "10 grains of rhubarb with 30 grains of magnesia duly mixed and taken in the morning while fasting, and repeated if necessary on the same day." His condescension is difficult to read today, but in its own time would have gone unnoticed. He patronized Sophia, "Have you not forgotten these kind friends of yours. The shower bath . . . [c]ontinue in that," he recommended, "unless you perceive any ill effects, such as debility, cold contracted skin, diminished appetite, or long drowsiness." If these symptoms emerged, then she was to give it up. He wrote:

> I am glad you wrote me . . . it is one of the privileges of our profession to learn much of human suffering for it has been made our duty to try to relieve it. My impression in regard to your illness has always been that perfect recovery is to be looked for only in the slow but sure operation of time. Symptoms may be palliated, and much present comfort experienced by the use of means. But expression of pain will return, with less violence however and then new means may be necessary. I have thought you better of late than at any former time, & ascribe much of your present weariness, and reluctance at exertion—the rapid changes you experience and your occasional depression, to mere influence of the season. The best of us quail beneath this sin of fire, and this sky of brass.

In November of that same year (1828) he wrote again, stressing his sincerity and at the same time her role as the recipient of his experimental medicine:

> I cannot but grieve, and I do sincerely lament, that you are still so great a sufferer—there is much that is dispiriting to the physician in the failure of means to . . . there is every thing to express the patient in this ineffective effort of our art. Still in your case, there is so much patience, so much of supremacy of the mind over the organ that is supposed in some way to contain it, that disease has made no conquest, and an assurance comes with this conviction that eventually you must do well. You will hardly expect this soon. You will not look

for it in the occasional intervals of suffering you may enjoy. Thus to
give you any promise on which to rely, must be of longer continuance
and of most perfect occurrence than they have been, and it may be
even more that something of this science is taking place, and I will
join with all your friends in sincere joy when the time of the last pain
shall have arrived and past, and the remainder of life to you, shall be a
long and uninterrupted interval of suffering. But I am still dealing in
generalities. . . . A physician is the creature of detail, but more when
I cast in my mind all that I have heretofore recommended. . . . I have
nothing new to recommend.

Channing's long letter ends with moral advice about her happiness,
admitting that she had suffered from his prescriptions: "Be as happy and
gay as you can be. . . . After suffering, obey all my rules of diet and study,
and I feel assured you will ultimately triumph." The remarkable fact,
demonstrated by the archival evidence in her journals, diaries, and letters, but not corroborated by biographers, is the extent to which Sophia
picked up on the value of education, something urged by her sister.
Sophia seemed to have discussed her intellectual efforts with her doctor,
and his paternal condescension again put her in her place. He wrote,
"Speaking of study I recollect what you asked me the last evening I saw
you. You spoke of Italian, & I think I did not dissuade you from giving
to it some attention. After thinking more of it, it does not seem to me that
it can be injurious. You should begin with moderation, for the head like
a limb that has not been long used, is less apt to easy use, and a moderate
effort only may trouble it."[71]

In September of the following year Channing sent his own publication, a pamphlet, along with his letter, asking her to read and perhaps
comment editorially. The pamphlet probably was the reprint of a public
lecture. In 1830 he again addressed her "My dear friend," and his tone
is more level—less condescending but not without an element of self-
interest. In the letter, he complains about the weather in Boston as being
dull and dreary, but implied that Sophia would be spiritually above
noticing such trivia, because of her physical suffering. "You have been
so long a patient and cheerful sufferer, that I suppose you hardly notice
such accidents as storms, and that now in this dark and dull atmosphere,
the light burns so brightly within that everything beams with it. I am

paying you no compliment in all this, for to such a nature as mind, spirit, why should there ever come darkness & gloom? The mind must depart from its nearest & best interests, not in a sense contradict & oppose its own nature, when it gives its high and noble powers to the exclusive service of anything without it." His cousin, the Reverend Doctor Channing, he wrote, wanted to escape another Boston winter, "& spend all its months in the fine island of Cuba": this is the first mention of such a trip in their correspondence.[72]

Sophia's diaries demonstrate the extent to which she internalized and accepted the mixture of religious advice and medical opinion in her resignation to suffering. Her entries describe a life of headaches, weakness, and constant reading all day, every day, for most of the day. She read Shakespeare, the Bible, and philosophers recommended by her sister Elizabeth, and she painted and drew and wrote letters, most of them from her bedchamber, sometimes while she was in bed. She recorded excerpts from her reading and from sermons she had heard, all mixed in with advice from her sister about what to read next, and advice from her doctors about how to relieve her fatigue. By far the most important passages in these diaries are those in which she has internalized the vernacular of the preachers she has heard, and the reading she has done, and delivers a sermon to herself, just as if she were pantomiming Dr. Walter Channing.

She advises herself about how to endure, and why she does so. She writes:

> I am just as tired as when I went to bed. . . . I shall soon be initiated into the secret charms of weariness. Patience . . . Patience is divine. . . . The greater the struggle, the more glorious the victory. Be Grateful for such occasions for proving your strength of soul. Let the body go. It will soon be laid low in the dust.
>
> Sunday 26th April . . . I began to take quinine today. . . . Sometimes it seems to me as if my life was a pathway of peculiar beauty— flowers springing with ever more loveliness, and indefinable atmosphere of music, a mingling of all bird voices floating around. Glimpses of endless vistas where is heard the distant falling of fountains, and sighing of leaves—a sky like a wide rainbow at one moment picturing 'city within city far withdrawn' at another a soft shadowing

& commingling of all colours in a plain, peaceful canopy of inexpressible beauty—that smile of our heavenly Father's parented Love almost visible & a tuneful hymn of praise from all inanimate & animate nature almost audible—this is always my life if left to itself.[73]

During this time, Dr. Walter Channing was a regular guest in the home. Sophia wrote to herself in her diary, "Dear Dr. Walter came home with us & staid till nine—as agreeable every moment of the four hours as it was possible. . . . He read over the lesson in the Old Testament . . . he said [it] was written for him & me, poor suffering mortals in this vale of sin," and then that weekend went to hear Reverend William Ellery Channing preach.[74]

In the ongoing illness, she continued to meld spiritual talk with excerpts from sermons she had heard and read, and the whole became a type of domestic advice book on moral character. She reported into her diary a headache, "overstretched nerves," and a "toothache." Her pain was so intense she feared to move because she would "bring back the pain in the brain regions." As she lay suffering in her bed, her sister Elizabeth (Betty) read to her the Reverend Doctor William Channing's sermon to raise her spirits. She then copied his sermons into her commonplace book, and when invited to take tea with Dr. Walter Channing, wrote that "it was a pleasure and a privilege."[75]

On "Sunday the 22nd," she wrote again about hearing the preaching of the well-known William Ellery Channing, and she thought him "thrillingly eloquent." Paraphrasing the sermon just heard into her diary, she recorded that "he emphasized that 'religion was natural'" to humankind, though many were taught incorrectly to think that it was not natural." Then she recorded that the preacher himself visited, mirroring the same moral messages of his physician cousin. "Dr. Rev. William Channing" visited, and "after quite a pause in the conversation . . . said "'Miss Sophia,' upon which I roused me & looked at him; but his face was buried in his hands, & so I waited for what should follow. He went on to say he had been reading about some females who would be painters & that it was said they were generally wanting in strength or as Fuseli said, 'There was no fist in it.' I tried to respond to his very kind notice of little me, but I found that no thought could find expression, & so I sunk away into my shell again."[76]

Though Sophia's neurasthenic condition was similar to that of many women invalids of the mid-nineteenth century—we might even go so far as to say "representative" of a certain class and category of patients—her diaries left a record of what one patient felt like under heroic cures administered by the most eminent, highly trusted physicians. Many others suffered in silence, and one only can conjecture about the level of fear about medicine that prompted so many Americans to seek alternatives, or to follow the latest quackery, whether herb or wheat, water or mind cure.

THE INVALID TOUR

When all other attempts at a cure had been tried, many physicians recommended that genteel invalids escape the Boston winter and go to Cuba. Dr. Walter Channing was following conventional medical practice in prescribing that Sophia do so. The first nineteenth-century record of an American invalid traveling to Cuba was written by Dr. Abiel Abbott (1828); it was published posthumously; he died on shipboard returning to New England. From the winter of 1833 through the spring of 1835, Sophia lived on the plantation of Dr. Robert and Laurette de Tousard Morrell. She continued to study, paint, and write voluminous letters home, but she also regained her strength and health. Once free from the prescriptions of arsenic and mercury, she rode her horse daily, observed everything in the natural landscape of Cuba from a transcendentalist perspective, and recorded the life among slaves with sympathy and interest.

Her host Dr. Morrell, himself sickly, managed a lucrative medical practice catering to the invalid trade, especially from transcendentalist Boston: he owned three plantations in Cuba run by slaves. His wife was the daughter of A. Louis de Tousard (1747–1817), vice consul of Philadelphia and New Orleans (c. 1811–1816), and her sisters were equally prominent women in Philadelphia and Paris. The journal is a rich historical document about prominent New Englanders and their engagement with the slave trade in Cuba.

Sophia's long letters home were shipped from Cuba at no little expense, to her sister Elizabeth in Boston (then working for A. Bronson Alcott) in care of her brother George, employed at Searle and Upham. Elizabeth circulated the letters among at least twenty-five eminent Bostonians, including Alcott, George Emerson, the chief justice of the State Supreme Court, Rev. William Ellery, and Dr. Walter Channing, Rev. F. W. P. Greenwood, and ten other prominent families, including Ralph Waldo Emerson's. She also held reading parties as long as seven hours. After Elizabeth popularized the letters in Boston, they were sent on to Salem, to Mr. and Mrs. Nathaniel Peabody. There Sophia's mother, with an even more meager learning than her daughters, set about cutting out and copying the letters for possible suitors. For example, if a passage about the slaves that Sophia found interesting was offensive, the entire page would have been rewritten. The remaining original pages, cross written to conserve paper, plus those rewritten by family members as they wished, were bundled together into three volumes, hand-sewn and bound, with leather spines, paperboard covers, and gold embossed titles on the spines, *Sophia Peabody's Cuba Journal.* It was a homemade book, the result of sickness and the interpretation of spirituality in recovering from ill health.[77]

When she returned to New England after the three-month stay in Cuba, her journal was given in 1866 to her suitor, later her husband, the novelist Nathaniel Hawthorne, as proof of her literacy and suitability to become a wife. He called her "The Queen of Journalizers," and she served throughout their twenty-two-year marriage as his amanuensis. The *Cuba Journal* is entirely typical of female travel writing in journals and diaries of the era, where little happened, but pages were filled with ink to describe its consequence, some of them written and crosswritten to save paper. Sophia's journal is about the daily life of an invalid on a plantation, but it is also the spiritual history of a soul. The *Cuba Journal* project, something of a homemade family scrapbook in letters, was written as an extension of her homeschooling by her elder sister Elizabeth and the leading transcendentalist luminaries. Sophia's immersion in the spiritual language of the sermons of Channing, and in the ideas inherent in transcendentalism, a study that had begun in her sick room, fill the romance of her interpretation of the natural. The letters she wrote are imbued with the atmospheric sunsets and glorious sweetness of nature that would have appealed to her transcendentalist audience, and they are self-conscious in that regard, and tellingly so, because she aimed to please her readers. She imagined herself into a romantic tale where Nature healed the ills endemic to her constitution. Her husband

Nathaniel, whom she later called "my lord and worship" when he entered their home in the evening, admired the *Cuba Journal*, and patterned one work of fiction, "Rappacini's Daughter," on her letter describing the Night Blooming Cereus. For example, she wrote, "Day, upon the threshold of the east Treads out the lamps of night," quoting Shelley, and continued, "said Sophy as she put her head into an atmosphere of gold this morning—& very soon she was pacing down the avenue in the full tide of splendor—Oh the flower of flowers! [about the night-blooming cereus] The convolvuli gave a purple expression to the lime hedge as far as I could see & riding along by that line of palms. . . . I wonder why some one does not build a house in this country & have its roof supported by fully grown palms! . . . Do you not think it is the ideal of a house!"

Later in her life, after their long marriage and raising their children, after Nathaniel had died, Sophia was again in ill health. In the year 1865 she had been recently widowed, and her perennial winter cough that would lead to her death in the next several years had reoccurred. She lacked money for fuel in the cold Boston winter. Her husband's publisher, James Ticknor Fields, had asked her to write a biography of her late literary spouse, but she did not feel strong enough to do it, so she settled into editing his voluminous notebooks instead. By the winter of 1866, a project she began out of sentiment took over her life. Deeply happy and contented to revisit her life with her children and her husband, whom she called her "Gorgeous Flower of Time," she was soon copying from nine in the morning until midnight, copying steadily about twenty pages a day, "driven by some sort of iron necessity," she wrote to her friend Annie Adams Fields, "taking time out only for a walk to the post." She wrote to the publisher that she had mastered the art of leaving herself out of the manuscript, a departure from her earlier habits, but in the next page exploded that she had "lost my head copying the Old Manse Journal—all the heavenly springtime of my married life comes back . . . so rich and delicate . . . and what I cannot copy is sweeter than all the rest." By the winter of 1867, Sophia was still working long hours and feeling the winter chill seriously, and doctors were expensive, she reminded her publisher. Nearly destitute and very ill, partially paralyzed and with her hair falling out, she was "aghast" to learn from Fields that she had already spent the ten thousand dollars he had advanced for her transcription and in addition owed him seven hundred dollars. Worried about her insolvency, she was still busy correcting proofs while trying to sell her home. After she had spent all the copyright income, Fields offered her 12 percent rather than the 15 percent royalties usually given to her husband. Sophia became hysterical, offering to give the publisher the Norway Spruce trees on her property if he would pay her "as much money as he could" for the edition of her husband's notebooks. When she later finished the project and sold her home, she moved to Dresden, then London, where, after another bout of influenza, she died in 1871.[78]

After so much grief, though, and so profound a loss of her "gorgeous flower of time," she must have looked out of that parlor window of the home she was trying to sell, where she once had used her diamond to etch into the glass, "Man's Accidents are God's Purposes," and had to resign herself to her suffering. Sophia's complete absorption in the religious language of her mentors, and her acceptance of Dr. Walter Channing's prescriptions about her study habits and emotional outlook as well as her health, are representative of the type of belief common among nineteenth-century women, whose compliance with the mix of religion and medicine contributed to the fused identity and cultural authority of the doctor and preacher.

But Sophia's lifelong meekness and obedience to all types of cultural authority, and her religious and physical submission also gave her something in return. It assured her social acceptance as a literate and spiritually sound female; it restored her to a place in the domestic order, when she had for so long been confined upstairs until she left for Cuba. Acceptance of medicine, failures and all, required a temperament of submission to God's will in the experiments and accidents of medicine, what Oliver Wendell Holmes had called the "topography of ignorance," but it also required a larger cultural understanding about domesticity and moral character and a deep resignation about the very few economic choices women had. Realistically, for any woman to have resisted the social authority of medicine and religion in the mid- to late nineteenth century would demand a courage that a romantic like Sophia Peabody simply could not have imagined.

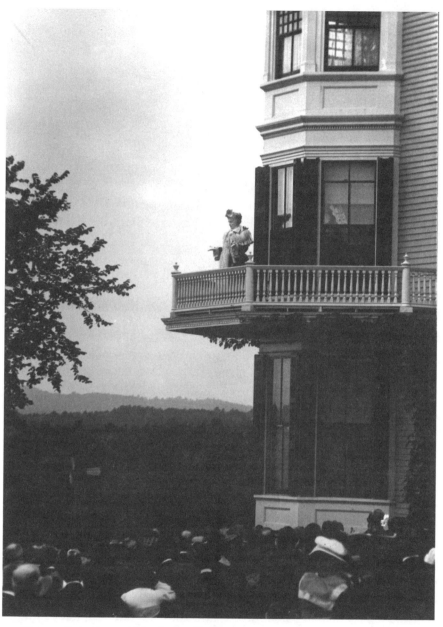

Figure 2.1: Rev. Eddy formally dressed in Victorian attire, on the second-floor balcony of her Pleasant View Farm in New Hampshire, addressing an assembled crowd, which routinely gathered on her lawn. Photograph, ca. 1901. Courtesy of MBE Collection.

Chapter 2

LAUNCHING A SCIENTIFIC RELIGION
CHRISTIAN SCIENCE AND THE BOOK

Who shall say I am not the happy genius of my household?
—William Carlos Williams, M.D.

Though Mary Baker Eddy was long-lived and had a foothold in both the nineteenth and twentieth centuries philosophically, she and Sophia Peabody Hawthorne were contemporaries in many respects—particularly in matters of health. But Mary Baker rejected what Sophia Peabody had accepted about medical authority on faith, the conventional thinking among Dr. Walter Channing and his Harvard Medical School contemporaries about what God intended for women as a rationale for their suffering, and the mix of religious speech and medical discourse that kept women in their place. The hardships of life as a woman three times widowed and a single mother no doubt made Mary Baker mature into as fierce a realist about medicine as she would be about religious principles, based on convictions about the power of healing through prayer and her personal experiences of the attitudes among the medical establishment about women's health in the nineteenth century.

Mary Baker Glover Patterson Eddy (1821–1910), founder of the Christian Science (CS) religion, was a woman of the nineteenth century without knowing anything of Margaret Fuller's feminism, Elizabeth

Peabody's idealism about female education, or Elizabeth Cady Stanton's biblical revisionism. She was a woman of the twentieth century in the sense that she possessed skills in organizational leadership, and in the sense that she intuitively understood what would become the popular language of modernity, media relations, and book publishing in order to build a reputation and manage its visibility among the people. This chapter is a profile of Eddy's rational, scientific approach to religion, one that incorporated the examples of Christ healing and framed an examination of widely accepted experimental practices that passed for regular medicine. In doing this she not only launched a science of mental religion, but built a worldwide organization through progressive management of all types of media, including news and books, methods accepted as routine in publishing and publicity today.

Eddy harnessed the ideas of the late nineteenth and early twentieth century that elevated the mind—ideas of Darwin, Freud, and later William James—and incorporated those intellectual currents that informed much of the popular consciousness of the late Victorian era, which would frame popular attitudes about science and religion into the early twentieth century, including Mind Cure and New Thought religions. Her admirers outnumbered her critics, but she had an abundance of both. Many of her seventy-five biographers praise her "prophetic" powers as they have written from within their own ideological frame. The "prophet" moniker is a stretch, though, in a life complicated by four marriages, one biological son she relinquished to foster parents, another son she adopted when she was sixty and he was forty-one and unmarried, several high-profile lawsuits, accusations of plagiarism, and enemies in the press as powerful as Joseph Pulitzer.

Her ideas about healing grew from her own empirical evidence, her experience of material medicine, and a spiritual intuition cultivated from a devotion to biblical reading. Her early life was typical of many New Englanders at the time and was comparable to Sophia's but without the educational advantages of New England transcendentalists in Concord, Massachusetts. Yet Mary Baker responded to the religious ethos and cultural expectations as a realist rather than a Romantic.

Baker grew up on a New England farm. Death and illness shaped the quality and character of her family life, as it did for many others during this period of American history, Not unlike other young women, Mary Baker struggled to regain her full strength after a girlhood during which she was physically weakened by illness, which meant for her the same bleak future as it did for many women, a life of limitation and confined domesticity. In the Baker family, where Mary was the last of six children, she was a "neurasthenic," the genteel invalid in her early years who received a dim prognosis from physicians about the likelihood of her ever leading a full life. She died at the age of ninety-one after a long and vigorous life, not because of doctors. Rather, she argued, it was because of the therapeutic power of prayer.

Even as a young women she resisted the inevitability of suffering that doctors thought was morally beneficial for women in her own day and culture. She made it her life's work effectively to oppose the types of heroic cures that Sophia Peabody Hawthorne endured, though the women never knew one another. Practicing material medicine was, in her opinion, "but a series of experiments—conjecture, doubt and dismay fill the minds of its most skilfull [sic] practitioner."[1] Since Christ never used drugs to heal in the Bible, Eddy questioned the morality of their use, as well as their efficacy: "The divine Mind never called matter medicine, and matter required a material and human belief before it could be considered as medicine. . . . Mind is the grand creator, and there can be no power except that which is derived from Mind. . . . Inferior and unspiritual methods of healing may try to make Mind and drugs coalesce, but the two will not mingle scientifically."[2] She responded to the failure of regular doctors, as well as to the prevalence of quackery, to construct a religion that would offer people solid spiritual hope about their own health. As this chapter describes, she built her own "brand" of religion based on prayerful rejection of regular medicine through publishing and the deft use of modern publicity practices.

An authentic spiritual seeker after biblical truth, Eddy had the capabilities of a modern CEO. A popular lecturer who attracted thousands to her Boston Mother Church and her Pleasant View farm in New Hampshire, at a time when medical quackery flourished and itinerant physicians trained as preachers often drew crowds, her organizational success did not escape hostile notice by the national press. A *New York Times* correspondent's death from pneumonia while under the treatment

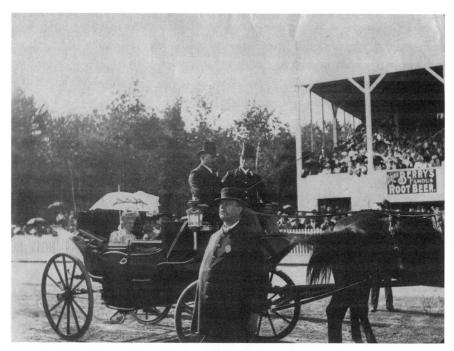

*Figure 2.2: Rev. Eddy at the New Hampshire State Fair,
in an open carriage on parade. Photograph, ca. 1900s.
Courtesy of MBE Collection.*

of a Christian Science healer precipitated numerous "strongly worded" editorials carrying headlines such as "Faith-Cure Murders" and "Manslaughter by Christian Science" that blazed across the pages of the national press. Charges of manslaughter and medical malpractice were brought against Christian Science practitioners who failed to achieve a cure, especially if it involved children. But failures of any type raised larger ideological questions about whether or not a Christian Scientist should be prosecuted for murder or malpractice, as a physician would be under the laws of jurisprudence, or whether "cheap martyrdom might strengthen them," as one journalist writing in opposition to the movement thought.[3] A British medical journal charged that Christian Science had contributed to the temperament of an age where there was "a jumble of pseudo science and irreligion." "Faith-healing . . . is a money-making concern," physicians charged.[4]

Eddy was realistic, especially about all that shaped the public perception. "Because divine Science wars with physical science . . . the old schools still oppose it. When the Science of being is universally understood, every man will be his own physician," she wrote in her foundational text for the religion, required reading for all believers, yet her words echoed the homeopathic domestic advice books so popular in her day.[5] What Christian Science proposed as original was a biblically based approach to physical healing through prayer, a "science" or discipline about health. "The ancient Christians were healers. Why has this element of Christianity been lost? Because our systems of religion are governed more or less by our systems of medicine. . . . The schools have rendered faith in drugs in fashion, rather than faith in Deity. . . . Material medicine substitutes drugs for the power of God—even the might of Mind—to heal the body."[6]

Among the more than seventy-five biographers of Eddy in the twentieth century, Robert Peel, who also wrote editorials for the *Christian Science Monitor*, was an astute chronicler. An intellectual historian, he saw Eddy as someone who epitomized the meaning of cultural resistance, though he did not use the term. Oddly, there is no evidence that as a young woman Mary Baker communicated or associated with the feminists of the nineteenth century, though she was in her later years on personal and familiar terms with both A. Bronson Alcott and Ralph Waldo Emerson, whom she tried to heal through prayer when he was near death. In Peel's view, Eddy represents what Basil Ransom in Henry James's *Bostonians* called the force of "damnable feminisation" that Peel astutely concluded is the epitome of what the term "cultural resistance" means. Peel wrote, "The genteel female of the period had turned subversive; she appeared on the one hand to be covertly imposing on society the standards of false gentility which, in the first place, it had imposed on her, and on the other hand to be overtly breaking out in a graceless feminism which brazenly challenged the male on his own ground."[7]

Yet her cultural resistance came not from any brazen political argument but from a submission to what she called Divine Will. In the vernacular of classic literature of Christian discernment, she built her "interior castle" on the discipline of prayer and constructed an alternative reality in such a way that authentic seekers who wanted to could live in the hope that the healing power she had experienced might be available to all. On balance, even humorists like Mark Twain, who called her "Eddypuss," admired her organizational talents, though he criticized her writing mercilessly. Other humorists working for magazines and newspapers also saw in the current religious climate at the turn of the century opportunity for satire and for sales.[8]

After the age of forty, Eddy established a biblically based healing religion and network of churches throughout the country through public lecturing and the media, a metaphysical college, a publishing company, a monthly international house organ, and a national newspaper. During this time she wrote and published more than two hundred revisions of the religion's foundational text, *Science and Health*. Rev. Eddy's modernity lay in her intuitive understanding that modern religion would use science—that is, Spirit and Psyche, or what she called Divine Mind—and would converge in and through popular religious culture in unprecedented ways, and that she would need media to propagate truth and disseminate information globally.

Her ideas about science and religion articulate attitudes resulting from the convergence of scientific and religious thought in the nineteenth century. According to medical historians, the many ideas about cosmology that followed Darwin's *Origin of the Species* (1859) contributed to the development of mind-cure therapeutics.[9] The writings of Christian evolutionists such as Henry Ward Beecher and Lyman Abbott, of theists like John Fiske (*Studies of Religion*, 1902) and Joseph LeConte, and the evolutionary cosmology of Henry Drummond's *Natural Law in the Spiritual World* (1883) and *Ascent of Man* (1894), contributed to the popular impetus among nineteenth-century writers to throw off materialism and "seek a new reconciliation of science and religion."[10] Yet her convictions about her own truth came from personal and empirical experience of the failure of material medicine to heal, and the failure of popular religion to solve the problem of human suffering. "Science represents a moral and spiritual force, which holds the earth in its orbit," she wrote.[11]

She liked to quote scientist Louis Agassiz, who had said that every new scientific truth went through three stages: first, people objected "that it conflicted with the Bible"; second, they claimed it had already been discovered; and third, they claimed they knew it all along.[12] Throughout

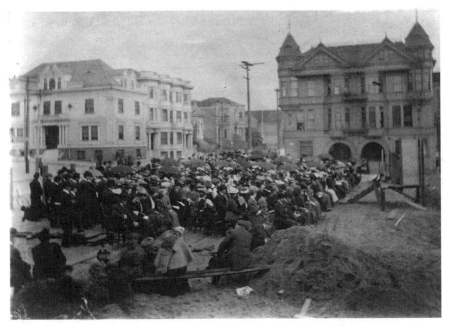

Figure 2.3: Christian Science service held outside after the San Francisco earthquake. Photograph, 1906. Courtesy of MBE Collection.

her life, she had to reassert at times her "discovery" of the Christian Science religion, her sanity, her ability to write original materials, and her right to the profits of the global publishing success of her key text, *Science and Health*, which by the turn of the twenty-first century was in its 246th edition, with runs of about one-thousand copies each. Animosity against her grew as Christian Science became more popular, celebrated by believers writing in the press. Hamlin Hill noted that between 1899 and 1909, "Well over a hundred articles about Christian Science appeared in magazines and journals, according to Reader's Guide," and "most were serious descriptions of or apologies for the religion."[13]

SUFFERING

Sophia Peabody's eldest sister Elizabeth, a leading educational reformer in Boston, was among the many self-educated women who sought better health through what would today be called alternative medicine. In the nineteenth century that meant hydropathy (water cures) and homeopathy, along with healthy foods, exercise, botanical medicine, and "mind-cures" such as mesmerism and animal magnetism, based on hypnotism. Homeopathy claimed that diseases "were simply dynamic or spiritual disturbances" that could be healed with the spiritual essence of medicines. "The magnetic influence of the homeopath's hand, along with the "imponderable essence of the drug" produced remarkable effects on disease, according to Jaller.[14] Among many other people in New England relying on homeopathy rather than the toxins, heroic cures, or standard medical practices was the young Mary Baker.

According to her most recent biography, published in 1999 by Radcliffe College, written by Professor Gillian Gill, a young Mary Baker Glover, widowed after six months of a first marriage and pregnant, endured a hard childbirth in 1844 that debilitated her in unknown ways for the remainder of her life. In the short term, her ill health forced her to make decisions she would live to regret. When she gave birth to her son George Glover II (1844–1915) in September 1844 and "fell desperately ill," Mahala Sanborn, a domestic servant of the Baker family, took care of both mother and child, giving the child to a wet nurse. Between 1845 and 1850, according to Gill, the boy was in the care of his mother and her family as she continued to struggle financially and physically. Impoverished, she tried to make a living first in journalism, where the local newspaper printed a few of her works, and then for a very short time she maintained a small school for children, and "failed to make much money" from either. For the next four years, Mary Glover tried to publish her poetry and essays in newspapers, with limited success.[15]

When her mother died and her father remarried soon after, Mary could no longer rely on her family's support. So in 1850, when her nearly forty-year-old servant Mahala also married, to a reportedly mean-spirited man named Russell Cheney, they took the six-year-old George into their home. Gill conjectured based on historical evidence that they did so because the boy was expected to be helpful on their farm, and "no doubt a sum of money" was involved. Gill wrote that it is a measure of how much the Baker family "disliked the boy and disparaged his abilities that they were prepared to give him into the care of mean-minded, unsuccessful, uneducated Cheney." George was "regarded as an indentured servant" because New Hampshire law at the time "permitted it," according to Gill.[16]

Based on archival evidence, and on information from the numerous biographers and the hagiography of the twentieth century, it seems that Mary Glover experienced a normal degree of maternal affection for her son, and only the circumstances of poor health and impoverishment forced the separation between mother and son, one exacerbated by the Cheneys' move to Minnesota six years later. It would be a good twenty years before mother and son saw each other again, and one must conclude that this, too, must have been a source of suffering.

About her struggle to regain her health, as a girl and then as a new mother, Eddy later wrote, "I wandered through the dim mazes of material medica, till I was weary of 'scientific guessing,' as it has been called. I sought knowledge from different schools—allopathy, homeopathy, hydropathy, electricity, and from various humbugs—but without receiving satisfaction. I found in the two hundred and sixty-two remedies enumerated by Jahr, one pervading secret; namely that the less material medicine we have, and the more Mind, the better the work is done; a fact which seems to prove the Principle of Mind-healing." Before developing a scientific and religious approach to healing, she first regarded homeopathy as the lesser of two evils: she regarded her own religion as a "step up" from homeopathy.[17]

Phineas Parkhurst Quimby (1802–1866), the clockmaker who became well known in New England for his use of animal magnetism, was one of several men whose "ghost" seemed to plague Eddy throughout her lifetime, even long after he died.[18] After too enthusiastic an initial intimacy, she devoted a great deal of energy for the rest of her life to distancing herself from him, especially as her critics alleged that she had "lifted the principles of Christian Science" from his writings, which she had edited and popularized. When Eddy first met Quimby in 1862, she had been searching for healing. Turning to many sects and fashions, she had ended her three-month stay at a hydropathy resort in upstate New York, which had done little to improve her health. So she put herself under the care of Dr. Quimby, whom she called a "magnetic" physician. "He used no drugs," she later wrote. "He did not pray for me when treating me: he talked with me on various subjects, then wet his hands in water and manipulated my head . . . but failed to cure me. He had almost no book learning, but advanced views on his subject of magnetic practice."[19] She regained her strength enough to recover from her various inexplicable ailments for awhile, and "maintained a small homeopathic practice" until she became "disenchanted" with homeopathy.[20]

During her experience of homeopathy in the 1850s, Mary Baker first observed what doctors today call the placebo effect, which had a significant impact on her later ideas about science and health and the power of religious belief to bring about healing. On this point, increasing numbers of physicians today are in agreement: that belief plays a pivotal and significant role in healing. As she administered increasingly smaller doses of increasingly diluted drugs, according to homeopathic practices, she observed how people continued to improve at the same rate whether they actually received the medicine in minuscule amounts or if they only thought they had.[21] This conclusion suggested that it was the power of belief in the medicine that brought about a cure, and it was belief that proved far more instrumental in patients' abilities to recover than the actual medicines themselves. Later, she described her experience as having "attenuated a grain of aconite till it was no longer aconite, then saturated some sugar of milk with a drop of harmless solution, and with the self same sugar have produced powerful perspiration. . . . The highest attenuation we ever attained was to leave the drug out of the question and administer it in the name of the drug, and with this original dose we cured a severe case of dropsy."[22]

In her correspondence during the 1860s with Dr. Quimby, Eddy's tone sounds reminiscent of the worshipful language in Sophia Peabody's letters to her physician Dr. Walter Channing. Also not unlike Sophia's relationship with Channing, in much of the correspondence between Mary Baker Glover and Quimby, it is hard to learn exactly what her physical ailment was about, except that she wanted the constant company of and attention from the doctor.

In the twenty-first century, the only thing that seems more antiquarian than house calls is the idea of writing a letter daily to one's physician requesting house calls. As Mary's persistent correspondence with Quimby demonstrates, she held him in high esteem—at least on first acquaintance: "My explanations of your curative principles surprises people! Especially those whose minds are all matter are convinced by the external appearance of errors . . . as for instance, the sores that have visited me, and yet I never lost my faith, or cursed wisdom, but have lived to receive all with usury again." But as her ill health persisted, her initial enthusiasm waned and belief in him gave way to pleading: "When I returned I ate just as the family did, and the three meals of rich food added to the fatigue of my journey revived the old error that such things hurt me. . . . The habit is yet so strong upon me that I need your occasional aid. . . . Please come to me to remove this pain and tell me your fee."[23]

In March 1863, Mary complained in a letter to Dr. Quimby about her nephew's drinking and smoking, and how his actions caused her not only untold "suffering from my old habits . . . pain in the back and stomach," but had caused her to want to smoke. Undoubtedly, this fed her ideas about the power of suggestion, an idea that was popular and highly current at nearly every circus or traveling fair at the time. She wrote her physician, "Do pray rid me of this feeling."[24] And in the fall of the same year, she wrote, "come once a day until I am better. I have had little appetite, and not rested well nights for two weeks. Now my food distresses me, pain between the shoulders, and FAINTNESS at the stomach."[25] This period of intimate correspondence consisting of complaint and response with Quimby came to an end abruptly with his unexpected death.

After her beloved physician Quimby died, she did not have much to lean on but her Bible, when in the winter of 1866 Mary fell on the ice, "struck" her "back," and "was taken up for dead, came to consciousness amid a storm of vapors from cologne, cholruform [sic] ether, camphor. . . . The Physician attending said I had taken the last step I ever should."[26] Among the biographers and hagiographers in the twentieth century, her healing and recovery from this fall have acquired "mythic" proportions among believers, according to Gill, who is not a Christian Scientist. Contemporary critics doubted the story as "specious fiction" because her injuries were minor, and her recovery incomplete.[27]

Mary later wrote of the time as if she were Paul on the road to Damascus: "I gained the scientific certainty that all causation was Mind and every effect a mental phenomenon. My immediate recovery from the effects of an injury . . . that neither medicine nor surgery could reach . . . led me to the discovery how to be well myself, and how to make others so."[28] After this accident, during a period of three years' solitude, when she prayed and read, she found that the "Scriptures had to me a new meaning, a new tongue. Their spiritual signification appeared; and I apprehended for the first time, in their spiritual meaning, Jesus' teaching and demonstration, and the Principle and rule of spiritual Science and metaphysical healing. . . . I named it Christian because it is compassionate. . . . God I called immortal Mind. That which sins, suffers, dies, I named mortal mind. The physical senses . . . error and shadow. Soul alone is truly substantial. . . . Spirit I called the reality; and matter, the unreality."[29]

Once she had outgrown the psychological need for Quimby, she was able to formulate ideas that would later become Christian Science. In solitary prayer, she developed her own language about disease and the healing power of Christ. She determined, according to another recent biographer who was a Christian Scientist, "that physicians and clergy were both guilty of fastening on humanity the errors that needlessly bound them to disease," and further, "she had come to the conclusion that there was a discoverable science of healing underlying Jesus' cures," that because of this Christianity must be linked to science, that disease was an "error" of the human mind, that there is a fundamental polarity between "truth" and "error."[30] In 1867, when she was forty-six years old, the year after Quimby's death, Mary's independent life began in earnest. She established a school in Lynn, Massachusetts, "with only one student," by her own account, and began her lifework of establishing a religion built on the ideas of biblically based healing through prayerful connection with the Divine Mind, without drugs of any kind.

Though many in her own day were skeptical about the healing power of prayer, and the controversy continues today in American medicine and religion (as chapters 3 and 4 of this book describe), Mary's idea of the power of a mental science about prayer as an avenue to health are regarded in some quarters as being ahead of their time. Christian Scientists are known in our own day for the nontraditional attitudes toward medicine, avoiding prescription medications and vaccinations. In the popular press today, it is not clear how the Christian Scientist thinks about going to a physician, but it would appear that individual decision is more liberally accepted than it was in her day. Yet it was the toxicity of the doctor's prescription medicine that she resisted most strongly, and in an 1880 "Bill of Rights" that she drew up for a lecture at Hawthorne Hall, Mary declared that every American had the "right to choose what physician they shall employ, what method they shall adopt . . . or what means they shall use to improve themselves physically," just as they had the right to freedom of religion.[31]

Detractors and critics in the press later charged her with plagiarizing ideas from Quimby, but that is a specious argument, considering how the preoccupation with the mind-body relationship characterized many movements, sects, and popular fashions in medicines during the late Victorian era. This charge of plagiarism, though, is still repeated today, and some medical historians persist in reiterating it, without understanding the distinction between Eddy's healing and the work of her disciples, such as Emma Curtis Hopkins, who rebelled and broke with the Mother Church to start their own brand of Christian Science that was associated with Unity and New Thought movements.[32] One wrote that "Christian Science had the classic parentage of Plato, a lingering flavor of New England's Transcendentalism, the fervor of the Victorian's faith in science, and the Christian's fascination with metaphysics. . . ."[33]

A number of critics have questioned where Mary's ideas came from, since she seemed to have been relatively isolated from what today we would call popular culture, and based on evidence in her archival papers preserved at the Boston headquarters of the Christian Science religion, her schooling was limited, as education for women was rare at the time. Her ideas were a combination of religious intuition and empirical experience. It was in her experience of medicine and quackery that she was closest to the Zeitgeist of the era, not through her reading, which remained devotional. The doctor-editor relationship that characterized the Channing-Peabody household also held in the case of Mary Glover and Quimby. But she had served as Quimby's editor, just as the Peabody sisters had often done for the literary and religious lights of the day, including Channing and, in due course, Nathaniel Hawthorne. When Quimby was putting together his book, *The Science of Man*, where he discussed "principles which inform all matter," much of the language he used might have been hers originally.[34] Later, her critics would look at that book and find resemblances to her own thought and words, a resemblance in its full historical irony that came full circle to trap her. Such accusations only seemed to fire her yen for breaking free, inspiring an entrepreneurship not considered a feminine virtue in an era when compliance, meekness, and domesticity were praised. Though a comparative study of the two texts by Quimby and Eddy has been done by detractors and by supporters, it yields more tedium than enlightenment. A more instructive approach is to look at the style and method of Mary Baker Glover Patterson Eddy's own manuscripts, and at the historical commonplace of the period: that many women served as an amanuensis for great men, which is how many were educated and how they achieved influence.

For example, for a reply to her detractors titled "Mrs. E's History," Eddy coauthored the piece with her Harvard-educated secretary Calvin Frye (1845–1917). Frye graduated from Harvard in the same class with Ralph Waldo Emerson, and served Eddy from 1882 to 1910 variously as bookkeeper, spokesman, confidant, aide, and metaphysical physician.[35] In an undated manuscript (probably around 1900), it looks like the two had talked, that Frye typed a draft, and that Eddy revised his typed draft with pencil emendations. In the draft, a mix of both hands, she declares what she did and did not read, and noted how strict her father had been about what she read, even objecting to her reading the books brought by her brother after he finished college, books by Locke and Bacon, Voltaire, and Hume.

> I never read Laiebnitz . . . Confucious, Plato, Socrates, Decortes [sic], Kant, Fichte, Spinoza, Berkeley, Emerson, or H. Spencer nor Swendenborg's works until after I wrote *Science and Health* was published. Hence if my writings resemble theirs they have only the likness [sic] of truth to truth. . . . I never borrowed my system of Chris Science Mind healing from any author or individual. . . . I have obtained all that I know of the works of the above authors except Confucious & Emmerson [sic] from . . . my Encyclopedia out of sheer curiosity to know if I had uttered their views unconsciously . . . The Bible was my only text-Book for S. & H. In my life I never read a work on Buddhism, Theosophy, Pantheism or Occultism in my life and never intend to shall read one.[36]

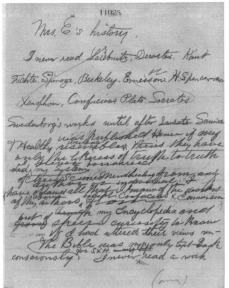
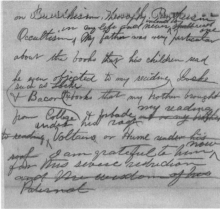

Figure 2.4: "Mrs. E.'s history." Autograph manuscript in the hand of Rev. Eddy, ca. 1900. Courtesy of MBE Collection.

Her critics charged that a woman was incapable of an original thought about religion and medicine. Though she made some errors in judgment about the character of her believers, she knew enough to surround herself with men who were more educated than she, and who believed in her religious sincerity and in the authenticity of her prayer life. The plagiarism charges against her lingered for the whole of her life, though she consistently refuted the charges in public lectures and in the newspapers. For a woman who wrote about herself in the third person in her Preface to the last edition of *Science and Health*, it would be consistent that in her media relations she would not sign her name to any refutation of such charges, but instead let others sign theirs, collaborating with them much as she did with Calvin Frye, who submitted their texts in draft form to her for her approval.

When the *Boston Post* had published an article circa 1883, which questioned pointedly "Who is the Founder of Mental Healing?" the pattern of using media to respond to detractors was established.[37] The style and habit of media relations, judging from the correspondence in the Eddy archives, was the following: to level countercharges against the latest pamphleteers, saying that they had not only lifted *their* ideas, but they were "ill educated," and to distance Christian Science from the imitators who were also founding religions and movements. Another letter charged one E. J. Arens (also spelled Erens), who had once been a student of "the late Dr. Asa G. Eddy and Mrs. C. E. Choate" of Boston, who now was in the business of publishing his own pamphlets (ca. 1880, 1881) "containing many pages taken from" the language and works of Mrs. Eddy on mental healing.[38]

The response in the Letters from the People column cut her former friend down to size in a way that Mark Twain would have admired.

> Dr. Quimby told us one evening, on our way to a lecture at the city hall in Portland, that he would exhibit some of his power to us in the hall. Accordingly, after we were seated, he said to us I shall set them to coughing, and immediately one after another commenced coughing until the assembly in general joined in chorus, longer or shorter, according to our directions. Then all of a sudden the coughing stopped but our laughter was not over, for immediately the people commenced sneezing as if a sudden choryzas had seized them, and pock[et] handkerchiefs were in quick requisition. . . . [His] method of treating the sick was manipulation; after immersing his hands in water he rubbed the head. . . . We asked him several times if he had any system . . . and he always evaded the subject. . . .[39]

And in another instance, she or those of her Publication Committee used their frontal-attack style of reply in the press to outline the theological principles of the faith:

> Christian Science has healed cases that I assert it would have been impossible for the surgeon or material medica to cure. Without Mind, man and the universe would collapse; the winds would weary, and the world stand still. . . . Human mentality, expressed in disease, sin and death, in tempest and in flood, the divine Mind calms and limits with a word. In what sense is a Christian Scientist a 'pest'? Is it because he minds his own business more than does the average man, is not a brawler, an alcohol drinker, a tobacco user, a profane swearer, an adulterer, a fornicator, nor a dishonest politician or business man? Or is it

because he is the very antipode of these? In what sense is the Christian Scientist a charlatan? Is it because he heals the sick without drugs?[40]

Yet the most often repeated boilerplate or stock reply for asserting the originality of the religious ideas was routinely followed by students who wrote on her behalf, asserting that *Science and Health* had been written over a period of eighteen years, and that Quimby owed his ideas to Eddy. On another occasion, Mrs. Eddy wrote to a student, Minnie B. Hall DeSoto, in September 9, 1886, offering her "hearty approval" for signing and publishing an article, commenting, "I have made some slight changes that will commend themselves to you. Ever Affectionately, M.B.G. Eddy/ Send me the enclosed article when printed." The student must have complied, because a copy of the newspaper article is in the clip file, and it reiterates that Christian Science is mental healing not "Mind Cure" or "Mental Science," and the article is signed by three students.[41]

In her many letters to editors of the leading newspapers of the day, Eddy addressed a broad range of theological and popular topics. To the *New York World*, for example, in reply to the question if faith in divine metaphysics were insanity, she wrote, "All sin is insanity, but healing the sick is not sin. There is a universal insanity which mistakes fable for fact throughout the entire testimony of the material senses. . . . The supposition that we can correct insanity by the use of drugs is in itself a piece of insanity."[42]

But unlike the New Thought and related movements, Rev. Eddy was a religious conservative whose beliefs were embedded in her "keys" to scripture. Though she did not enjoy a broad liberal education, she read the Bible intensively and prayed daily. By all accounts, even among her detractors, she was devout. Moreover, there is little in the religion she founded that heralds the freedom from doctrinal discipline encountered in the twentieth-century New Thought movement and related bohemian styles of free interpretations of scripture. Discipline, both mental and religious, was central to her religious views and to her interpretation of scripture, and the practice of prayer responsible for healing. Without the piety and the discipline, healing through prayer was impossible, she believed. Around 1888, as Harley's recent biography of Emma Curtis Hopkins observes, rebellious students like Hopkins, who had once been editor of the *Christian Science Journal*, broke away, set up their own churches or schools with the same or similar names, and wrote their own derivations of the science of healing. These breakaway groups contributed to the movement called New Thought, which extended to the New York literati and avant-garde between 1920 and 1940. Eddy often disciplined students through the church structures and governance, but by the time she grew old, she seemed to mellow on the point, and accepted the many imitators as beyond her control. In the Preface to her final edition of *Science and Health*, Eddy wrote that since the first edition of the book in 1875, "Various other books on mental healing have been issued, most of them incorrect in theory and filled with plagiarisms from *Science and Health*. They regard the human mind as a healing agent, whereas the mind is not a factor in the Principle of Christian Science. A few books, however, which are based on this book, are useful."[43]

EDUCATION AND WOMEN'S HEALTH

In 1881, Eddy established the Metaphysical College in Boston to educate Christian Scientist practitioners, graduating four thousand in the next eight years, by her own accounting. She advised "diseased people not to enter the class," because during the classes many had been healed, she wrote, and such students were poor scholars, because "the glad surprise of suddenly regained health is a shock to the mind; and this holds and satisfied the thought with exuberant joy."[44] The purpose of the college and of the religion was "spiritual formation, first, last and always. . . . Mortals must learn to loose their estimate of the powers that are not ordained by God, and attain the bliss of loving unselfishly . . . conquering all that is unlike Christ."[45]

Certain key women's health issues remain as politically divisive today as they were in the late nineteenth century. Childbirth was the chief threat to the public health of women. Though abortions were not unheard of, it was far more common for a woman to die from puerperal fever, the infection caused by the dirty hands of physicians, or from the brutalities of the medical practice of etherization and use of instruments. Nothing shaped women's health more in the late nineteenth century than childbirth, and probably in no other area of women's health were the practices of the medical establishment more ill informed, from the patient's perspective.

By January 1887, when the Christian Science Church had been established for more than a decade, and the Metaphysical College established for six years, the Rev. Mary Baker Eddy took up the highly controversial problem of pain in childbirth. Her college offered a course in obstetrics to a mixed class of both men and women advanced practitioners. Physicians like Channing had claimed that ether relieved the pain. Eddy had the audacity to claim that prayer freed women not only from the pain but also from the fear caused by "wrong thinking" about childbirth.

The idea of women's role as sufferer, as Dr. Walter Channing's book (discussed in chapter 1) epitomized, the idea that God had intended—indeed wanted—women to suffer, and the idea that the pain of childbirth "bonded" mothers to their offspring were all part of the mixed religious and medical rhetoric that Christian Science not only rejected but tried to set straight with advances in education about childbirth for women that might provide an alternative reality to their suffering. Mrs. Eddy's course in obstetrics, open to both men and women who studied anatomy in the same classroom, was a startling break from conventional approaches to medical training at the time. While the Rev. Eddy taught the theological part of the class, one man named Ebenezer J. Foster, M.D. (1847–1930), a forty-year-old experienced homeopathic physician, was brought in to teach the anatomy module of the classes. Within the year, Eddy had adopted him.[46]

As she replied to a prospective student interested in obstetrics who had written a letter to her that Eddy wanted to publish in the *Christian Science Journal*:

> I wish you would enter my next class in obstetrics, you and your husband. I have now a Student to assist me in this Class he will teach the mechanical and anatomical portions and I the metaphysical ones of this study. He has graduated at the Medical College of Philadelphia, been in practice 20 years and never lost a mother or child at childbirth. His practice was large and successful He is president of the Vt State Bureau of Homeopathy his name E. J. Foster.

According to the class notes for the obstetrics class, the anatomy discussion was not in any way unusual.[47]

Though she had been twice widowed and once divorced, she had outlived all her siblings. Mary Eddy's finances were in "good order" by 1888, when she adopted Ebenezer Foster, whom she called "Benny" and sometimes "darling." According to his neighbors, as recounted by Professor Gill, E. J. Foster was a "womanish" sort of man, effete, unmarried with no children, happy to praise and delicate in his flattery.[48] Eddy's rapid affection for him alarmed her closest associates in the association. He soon moved in and lived without charge in her home, accompanied her on a highly publicized lecture tour to Chicago in 1888, and said "yes" when she offered to adopt him in October of that year. She gave him positions of importance in the organization, and entrusted to him the title of president of the Mother Church, though not the prestigious title of First Reader.

The tone of one of his letters to Mary Baker Eddy on July 4, 1893, when he was forty-six years old, the year before they parted ways, speaks volumes about the style of a buttery man:

> My Dearest Sweetest Darling Mother,
>
> This morning all the people of the country seem to be turned to any thing but Good, Spirit, but my thought and my love goes out only to the dearest and most blessed of all the earth, my Mama! Who has brought true freedom to all the world. She and her work are only worthy to be celebrated. The world shall some day know her worth and sing her praises through Love. Five years ago to day I came to you and to day my love and gratitude are five times stronger and purer for you my blessed Mama. My choice would have been to be with you to day, but where ever I am I want to make a days march nearer Spirit, Love. After my mornings work is done I shall commune with Good as much as possible the remainder of the day. . . . Benny.[49]

Certainly the adoption must have created conflict between her biological son and her adopted one. Writing to her son George in reply to his having sent pictures of her youngest grandchildren, George Glover III and Andrew Jackson Glover, she wrote that "I shall take more interest in seeing your . . . pictures, after you answer the letter that my adopted son wrote you long ago. 'Tit for tat'—is an old maxim, and *useful* when understood."[50] Both sons turned around and sued her for her wealth in the last years of her life, in what biographers refer to as "the Next Friends" lawsuit. In her will, despite their offenses, Eddy left $45,000 to Benny, and $245,000 to George, under the condition that he would not contest her will—which, in due course, he did.[51]

With the adoption of E. J. Foster-Eddy, not only had she made herself vulnerable to the public perception that her mind was unsound, but in her poor judgment had invited satire from humorists like Twain, who were glad to take advantage. In the short term this undermined the credibility of her religious accomplishments, and no doubt the validity of the Christian Scientists' public image based on faith healing. It also created more problems than necessary by providing fodder to the press, which looked at her from a purely secular standpoint. Members of the press needed to attract attention from readers. If they had to be irreligious to do so, they had a history of British and French caricaturists intent on deflating doctors' social status as precedent. Women preachers were a slow-moving target.

In the college she established, Rev. Eddy shrewdly did not challenge directly the medical establishment by trying to train midwives. She persisted in her position that Christian Science practitioners were neither midwives nor doctors, but offered the women a healing presence through prayer. According to one biographer, "The object was not to fit them to act as doctors or midwives, but to prepare them to cope spiritually with the various phases of 'false belief' connected with childbirth." She integrated testimonies of painless childbirth in her later editions of *Science and Health*.[52]

For those wishing to enroll in the obstetrics course, the Metaphysical College required prerequisites. As always, students needed to be in good health, and to have completed the primary and normal levels of the class and have practiced healing for at least one year. The primary class given to all who aspired to become Christian Science Mind-healers consisted of twelve classes over three weeks, costing aspirants three hundred dollars. The normal class was followed by the next level, with a two-hundred-dollar tuition, limited to practitioners with at least one year's experience, "certificates from their teachers, good health and moral character."[53]

If a practitioner had completed both the primary and normal course levels, the course in metaphysical obstetrics, which at first cost one hundred dollars, then was doubled almost immediately, probably because it required two instructors—one a homeopathic physician to address matters of anatomy, and also the teaching of Rev. Eddy about scripture. The obstetrics course consisted of six daily lectures and was restricted to graduates of the Metaphysical College.

Theology was the last required course (tuition: two hundred dollars). All tuition was paid in advance; husband-and-wife teams could enroll for the cost of a single student. One soldier who had been wounded in the Civil War wrote to Rev. Eddy asking for a reduction in tuition, and that his wife be allowed to enroll in the obstetrics class directly from the first level. She noted that the two could repeat the first level, which they had taken elsewhere for a combined tuition at a reduced rate (three hundred dollars), and after that, she would have to decide the matter of reduced tuition.[54]

But Eddy was treading on sacred ground and on thin ice when she attempted to bridge the difference between medicine and religion and women's suffering in childbirth. The newspapermen of the day no doubt waited for any breath of failure, and in due course, one celebrated case hit the headlines. Mrs. Abby H. Corner, a woman who had claimed falsely, it seems, to have been trained in the program, had assisted her daughter at the birth of her grandchild—and lost both. She was tried and acquitted. The Christian Scientist Association was quick to call her an imposter, and to point out that she had not been trained as an "accoucher," had only attended one term of the four-year required courses, and had not studied in the obstetrics course. "The West Medford Case, so far as is known, is the first instance of death at childbirth in the practice of Christian Science. This fact is of vital importance when compared with the daily statistics of death on such occasions caused by the use of drugs and instruments. Does their medical malpractice, and the mortality that ensues, go unnoticed because of their frequency?"

In language that would leave no doubt, the Christian Science Publishing Committee replied to her critics:

> Are the medical scoffers who sit in judgment on mind-healing willing to lift the veil on the charnel house for others to read the records

of their blunders and count the number of their victims. . . . All professions are subject to impostors, Christian Science included. But the history of science is by no means at the mercy of charlatanism. Recreant practitioners in any school of medicine are a disgrace to it. The mind curer, faith curers and mesmerists, who never touched the altitude of scientists, are reckoned among them all the same. The Globe reports that the leader of faith cure, Dr. Cullis, saying he always employs drugs, hygiene and material methods first, and God last in his practice. . . . Dr. Cullis admits that . . . God cannot deliver a mother in travail, for this is the proper province of drugs, the knife and the forceps.[55]

This attitude was the antithesis of the Christian Science theology that informed the teaching of obstetrics in the college; it characterized the thinking of the allopathic obstetricians from whom the Rev. Eddy set out to liberate suffering women.

Mary Baker Eddy's second lesson in the course raised interesting theological questions that would have been controversial at the time. Among the questions she raised with the class were: "Is conception spiritual?" "Would not wrong thoughts mark and mar the embryottic [sic] concept?" "Is suffering the normal condition of childbirth?" "How are the pains of childbirth destroyed?" "Did Adam give birth to Eve and was a surgical operation requisite at childbirth?" "Would not the true concept of being held firmly in the mind of the practitioner and presented mentally to the thought of the mother prevent the possibility of peril at childbirth?"[56] Explaining the theological infrastructure of her ideas about religion and health would occupy her for the rest of her long life.

By 1894, Eddy had dropped Foster-Eddy from the role of publisher because of his alleged affair with his woman secretary, a fracas that developed after a series of other problems. In trying to explain this strange relationship, Gill concluded that it was not that Mrs. Eddy needed an heir, but that Benny "spoke the current language of spirituality so fluently" and deceived her into thinking of him as a kindred spirit.[57] According to the church archives, what Mrs. Eddy took away from the ill-advised episode was to "see how her adopted son had always blamed his mistakes on the malicious thinking of others." After 1890, as the church continued to grow—and so, too, did the attacks against her—she determined not to blame her own mistakes on others, and to pray her way out "of the evil in these situations," and to divorce the attacks from the person who wrote them. She incorporated this in her advice letters to healers.[58]

Five years after the 1875 publication of the first edition of *Science and Health*, her estranged son returned. In 1879 George Glover II was thirty-five, wounded from service in the Civil War, "barely literate," married to an illiterate wife nearly two decades his junior, with too many children: the couple was in financial need and seeking economic backing. He accepted his mother's faith as his own but realized that she and her newest husband, Asa Gilbert Eddy, were in no position to help him financially.[59] Nonetheless, he continued his appeals for money until her death.

When Asa Gilbert Eddy died of a heart attack in June 1882, in her grief and emotional turmoil, the widow Eddy "declared that he had been killed by mesmerism, mental arsenical poisoning (MAM) directed upon him by her enemies," among them the rebellious student and plagiarizer, Edward Ahrens, whose attempts to compete with Mrs. Eddy had incensed her late husband, caused him to put in long hours, and probably contributed to his death.[60] Making public statements about the power of mind poisoning did Eddy's reputation no good as a foundress and leader of a religion based on science. But in a sense, according to today's mind-body medical standards, the enemies of Mary's fourth husband did indeed "kill him," given the stress and his preexisting heart condition. Probably there was little either could have done by that time. Eddy's accusations and manner of explanation, though, left her wide open for ridicule in the press, and later charges that she clung to the darkness of mind cure and mental suggestion.[61]

THE BOOK

Royal S. Copeland, a homeopathic physician who—as U.S. senator from New York helped create the Food and Drug Administration, changing the way people once thought about advertising prescription drugs as unseemly—once "conceded" that Christian Science "had beaten to a frazzle" homeopathy in terms of "organization, means of publicity, and popular success."[62] At the same time public attitudes were in flux about advertising and drugs, changes were occurring in how authors dealt with the biggest problem for writers in the nineteenth century: how to make a living from publishing books, and how to advertise and sell literary wares at a profit, bypassing booksellers if possible and reaching the reader directly. Mrs. Eddy not only built a newspaper business, but her success and profitability with creating the book *Science and Health*, without using booksellers and by reaching readers directly with a variety of new methods, contributed to how leading authors such as Mark Twain thought about book publicity.

In 1875, she published the first edition of what would become the foundational text for the religion, *Science and Health*, about 1,000 copies, at 456 pages, printed by W. F. Brown & Co.[63] The bibliographic provenance and printing history about this book are unique in American literary history, demonstrating the personal habits of the woman as a writer and editor. In a study of the textual changes in the 236 editions printed between 1875 and 1911, one author noted that many textual changes occurred in interim editions, and that the author was constantly making "clarifying alterations" in the language and fine points in the text. The eighty-fourth edition of the text was placed in the cornerstone of the Mother Church on May 21, 1894. Between 1875 and 1911 there were seven complete reprintings of the text, and numerous interim editions.[64]

Though a separate bibliographical study could be written about the reasons for all the changes to this foundational religious text, and what doubts and claims Eddy corrected in these revisions, no book in American history has undergone so many revisions. For example, her concordance to the Bible, called "Key to Scriptures," was added after the first edition. In this and the next edition, the word "Substance" was used as a synonym for God; Eddy stated her preference that God be rendered in the feminine gender.[65] The second edition, published in 1878 by Rand, Avery & Co., at 167 pages is called the Ark Edition, because its cover design included an illustration of an ark. Originally planned to be an edition of more than 500 pages, only 167 pages could be salvaged, because there were so many typographical errors. In 1881 a third edition, printed by University Press, John Wilson & Son, Cambridge, appeared in two volumes of 270 and 214 pages each, and this edition displayed the first use of the religion's logos, the Cross and Crown, not altered again until 1908.

In the third through fifteenth editions, "God" or "Spirit" is retained as feminine. In the sixth edition, in 1883, printed by University Press, again in two volumes, "Key to Scriptures" was added as part of the book itself, not as an addendum. In the 1886 sixteenth edition handled by University Press, the whole book was put into one 552-page volume. Rev. James Henry Wiggin (1836–1900) prepared a 38-page index, which was retained until the 226th edition.[66]

From the 1886 edition, Rev. Eddy approved one of three sentences to be placed on the walls of the church edifices: "Divine Love always has met, and always will meet, every human need." In the 1891 edition (the fiftieth), marginal headings were introduced and other refinements of presentation were printed. In 1902, the 226th edition included a new chapter, "Fruitage," and the author's revised marginal headings. The 1907 edition replaced the testimonials in "Fruitage" with more current witness statements by people who had been healed by reading the book. In 1910 Mrs. Eddy requested that her picture be removed from the frontispiece, in a continuing effort to put less emphasis on her personality, so that the religion would stand on its own after her death.[67]

As publisher of *Science and Health*, Ebenezer Foster-Eddy, in his heyday before his estrangement from Eddy, "made an excellent profit." The book retailed for three dollars, with forty-five cents spent on production costs: Mary Baker Eddy received one dollar, Foster received one dollar, and all advertising costs were covered by the association.[68] In Twain's book, *Christian Science*, published in 1907, but begun much earlier for *Cosmopolitan* magazine, his satire grew out of a comparison of his book profits with Eddy's. In his personal copy of Sir William Besant's *The Pen and the Book*, Twain scribbled into the margins comparing his own productions costs, royalties, and finances with Rev. Eddy's.

Twain alleged Eddy published *Science and Health* in continued revisions and reprintings, making a 700 percent profit. Twain wrote, "I am obliged to doubt that the three-dollar *Science and Health* costs Mrs. Eddy above fifteen cents, or that the six dollar copy costs her above eighty cents. . . . When the Supreme Being disseminates a saving Message through uninspired agents—the New Testament, for instance—it can be done for five cents a copy; but when He sends one containing only two-thirds as many words through the shop of a Divine Personage, it costs sixty times as much. I think that in matters of such importance it is bad economy to employ a wild-cat agency."[69] Twain did not make near that profit, even from *The Adventures of Huckleberry Finn*, and while he must have been envious, he was willing to learn from someone who kept rewriting the same book, for increasing profits, and who had no use for booksellers, but revised, reedited and reprinted the book as required reading for her members. The fact that a book could be a required product set Twain to thinking about production costs and profit margins.

Twain's marginalia on his copy of Besant's *The Pen and the Book* reveal the renowned humorist as competitive with and learning from the publishing success of Eddy's *Science and Health*. In the Besant chapter titled "Costs of Production," Twain responded to Besant's cost estimates with this comment: "Mrs. Eddy's 1,000 would cost $400 and sell for $4,375—just about ten times the cost." And in the section of that book where Besant advised about methods of publication, he again compared his own poor profits against his imagination of what Mrs. Eddy's were: "When 28,000 of MSS had been bound and delivered, (at 60 off to Gen Agents. Paid the pub 3 percent . . . I got $1.37 1/2 a copy & out of it paid 60 and 68 for manufacture, which was robbery. I cleared about 65c on 10,000 copies." Where Besant's estimates applied to second and third printings of the same edition, Twain wrote, "This would make the Eddy book cost $3,250 (say 32 c a copy) & sell for $43,750— something above 1,000 per cent profit." Where Besant estimated costs of types of book covers, Twain wrote, "double this for Eddy," "$900 for 2,000 copies cloth say 45c per copy or 550 per cent above cost." About advertising books, Twain wrote "Right" along the margins of Besant's comments that "advertisings do not by themselves cause a book to 'go'. The circulating libraries are far more useful than any advertising columns," a tactic Eddy used early on to promote knowledge about *Science and Health*.[70]

Twain's near-obsession with imagining Eddy's profits demonstrates how two authors dealt with the problem of marketing books and how, in bypassing booksellers and agents who siphoned off the profits, both the religion and the profits from the book increased. Mrs. Eddy didn't need booksellers because she could use the church congregation infrastructure to sell her book, and she relied on her followers to put the book in every local public library, spreading the reputation of the book through word of mouth.

Twain's personal suffering over the death of his young daughter is well documented, as are his financial struggles, so he must have looked on Rev. Eddy's popularity with mixed emotions. In his marginalia above Besant's chapter heading "The Method of the Future," Twain rated the difference between their books as commodities. "Nothing could be stupider," Twain scribbled in pencil, "than selling *unrequired* things by methods suitable to *required*—like salt, matches, tobacco &c. Selling books through booksellers is infinitely stupid. Thro' the PA, you offer the book *directly* to the man himself. And there should be a . . . postcard (salable @ 10 percent above its face) to be filled in as one coupon (addressed to himself by the sender?) with a 1/2 cent stamps on it. If you want a free, sell 5." And at the bottom of the page, Twain wrote, "I published Huck Finn—success. Pub'd 3 & paid pub a royalty—poor job."[71]

In 1883, Eddy started the *Journal of Christian Science: An Independent Family Paper to Promote Health and Morals*, an eight-page, three-column, bimonthly tabloid newspaper first printed on April 14, 1883. Doing most of the writing and editing herself at first, she was scouting for good writers, editors, and speakers to whom she could delegate.[72] Articles appeared over her own byline, but also included news items that demonstrated her theological and medical purposes, as well as her own and others' sentimental verse. Initially, there were four hundred subscribers, and by the fall of 1884 an additional one thousand to three thousand single issues also were being sold; by 1893, according to records, the *Journal* had fifty-two hundred subscribers.[73] She used the newspaper to disseminate the ideas promulgated in her sermons, writings, and teachings. "The theology of Materia Medica of Jesus were one," she wrote on the first page of the first issue: "Since God is supreme and omnipotent, Materia Medica, hygiene and animal magnetism are impotent," the Rev. Eddy declared, going on to argue that "true knowledge of God, imparts the only power to heal."[74]

Eddy's marketing and promotion of the *Christian Science Journal* between 1883 and 1910 established it as the national house organ for the religion. In a prospectus dated April 13, 1883, Eddy wrote that the purpose of the paper was "to bring to many a household hearth health, happiness and increased power to be good, and to do good. . . . We are needing funds to establish its permanent publication."[75] Advertising in the *Boston Sunday Herald* the day after the first issue appeared, Eddy urged all students of the religion "to take a personal interest in the *Journal* and put it into the hands of every patient."[76]

By January of the following year, though, it seems that the regular press had taken some notice of the house organ. Eddy wrote to one of her students, a businessman named Col. Eldridge Smith, whom she wanted to enlist to help her manage her publishing operations, that "the first magazines and newspapers in the land exchange with me their large weeklies and monthlies for my bimonthly folio."[77] On March 18, 1884, Eddy moved that the bylaws of the religion be amended to include a provision "that every member . . . subscribe . . . and obtain annually not less than six subscribers for it or forfeit their membership." In a few weeks, the statement was softened, but not by much: "or be liable to or forfeit their membership," a provision removed from the bylaws by the year's end, with the directive dated October 4, 1884, that "Perhaps it were well to correct the impression . . . that the appeal for aid in behalf of the *Journal* was made at the request of Mrs. Eddy herself."[78]

By August 1884, with Col. Smith on board as publisher, the *Journal* became a monthly publication, and within six months, he informed Eddy on May 6, 1885, that "subscriptions are coming in at the rate of 10 or 15 a day" as promotional materials were published in the *Boston Evening Traveller* and *Boston Evening Transcript*.[79] Also in December 1884, Eddy relied on using the *Journal* in California to promote the religion, and "to correct the false teaching and false practices in your state and abide by the text-book of the science "Science and Health." By October of the following year, an advertisement in the *Journal* urged students to help reach the goal of ten thousand subscribers.[80]

Silas Sawyer, manager of the Christian Science Publishing Society, asked all readers of the *Journal* in 1885 to make sure their local public libraries and reading rooms had recent copies. In early 1888, the *Journal* started promotional pricing and inserting order forms into the paper, and Eddy urged everyone to "take our magazine, work for it, and read it."[81] By June 1889 (through 1897), the newspaper was given over to the National Publication Committee, and a young businessman, William G. Nixon, was appointed publisher. Dropping incentives in October 1889 as something that was "wholly worldly," Nixon's zeal led him to write to Eddy that the Journal was "prospering" and he had new ideas about its promotion. He wanted to send personal letters to the religion's teachers and students, "and that your publications and those of the Society be the only literature recommended to those learners. Do you not think the time ripe for us to proclaim this Gospel through every respectable periodical that will hear us?" Then Nixon proposed that two thousand copies of an early version of her book be printed "with an 'ad' of the Society's publications on one cover, and those of Mrs. Eddy's works on the other, to be used for gratuitous circulation among strangers at the next national Association," and in order to boost sales of the Journal and Science and Health through "legitimate advertising," advertisements should be printed in the "St. Louis magazine" and Zion Herald of St. Louis (a Methodist paper). Nixon had other advertising and promotional ideas, but Eddy forbade it, alleging that his time spent in perpetuating "schemes" was unholy, that he was using "the means" that God has forbidden."[82]

Distancing herself from the publishing business in order to run the church, Eddy replaced Nixon with Joseph Armstrong, and E. J. Foster-Eddy was given the title of publisher of Science and Health. In May 1893, Joseph Armstrong commented to Eddy about the fifty-two hundred subscribers to the Journal. He wrote that "we ought to have 15,000" subscribers. As the publishing committee prepared for the Colombian Exposition, the Chicago World's Fair of 1893, plans were made to give away free copies of the Journal and bound volumes of Mrs. Eddy's writings. Subsequently, new subscription incentives were renewed in 1898, as were trial advertisements in the mainstream press, in periodicals such as the Century Magazine.[83] A month later, though, Rev. Eddy backed off from advertising her publications to those "whose hearts are not ready for Christian Science," and advised "drop advertising altogether except in our own ranks."[84]

By 1899 another newspaper, the Sentinel, was added to the roster of the religion's publications, which were receiving widespread distribution in the Washington, D.C., area and continuing to be dispensed to public libraries by the church's members. The church leadership advised all members "who can afford it" to subscribe to the organs. However, an editorial expressed disapproval of any attempt "to force CS literature upon 'unprepared thought.'"[85]

Rev. Eddy asked that arrangements be made with "leading papers and magazines throughout the country to place our periodicals on exchange with theirs." Within five years, that list numbered seventeen thousand.[86] This put Christian Science on a collision course with the press. Rev. Eddy's ability to organize well and to publish strategically put her in the precarious position of publicly sharing an "organ" intended for internal audiences. Predictably, this could bring trouble—and it did.

MEDIA RELATIONS

In addition to publishing the periodical and the book, which was in constant revision and use, Rev. Eddy needed someone to deal with the mainstream newspapers and tabloids, which always seemed to be on the attack. The individual had to be Christian in his manner, yet firm and socially adept with newspapermen and editors.

Alfred Farlow (1857–1919) served as manager for the Christian Science Committee on Publication between 1899 and 1914. His writing was clear and concise, as the press needed; his tone was always kind, as Rev. Eddy required.[87] Farlow closely monitored Eddy's public profile and had the job of replying to attacks in articles and in letters to the editor, most printed in the mainstream press. In his own words he kept "a pretty tight rein on things . . . pertaining to newspapers."[88] Farlow related the time when a bodyguard smashed the camera of a photographer who was taking an unauthorized, unposed photo of Mrs. Eddy. "As newspaper agent for the church it fell to me to heal the wound which had been occasioned." The photographer eventually became a leading editor-in-chief of one of the "great daily papers of the country," according to Farlow, so his time had been well spent.[89] The Committee on Publication defined its mission to "correct in a Christian manner" impositions on the public . . . injustices done Mrs. Eddy or members of this church by the daily press, by periodicals."[90] Farlow was considered "an excellent editor and writer," who took directions from Eddy and others on her staff. He advised one member to "tone down" criticism of doctors who did not believe in the ideas about medicine without drugs.[91]

Farlow instructed followers in Australia similarly: "Write them in such a way that the editor will not feel that he is whipped when he publishes your article."[92] Farlow's "excellent business tact," a requirement for the job, stood him well in his relations with newspaper editors.[93] Most of his relations with newspaper editors were face-to-face, and he learned to appreciate deadlines and space considerations. "I have associated myself with the editors and reporters to such an extent as to become one with them, and to be thought of by them as a newspaperman. I sit and chat with them, even listen to their yarns and laugh and joke with them. . . . I make them see that I am their friend and this serves as a barrier against the publication of things which they know are offensive to me. When I have a communication I take it to them in person . . . and they never go back on their word."[94]

When the usual criticisms about plagiarism were reprinted, Farlow tried to quash the rumors: "Dear Teacher; When I last conversed with you on the Quimby matter, you advised that I should not give it further notice in the press. . . . I am a little confused as to whether you really want me to give further notice to this matter. Like many other falsehoods they keep repeating it and unless we keep on correcting it, they say we have become convinced and therefore silent."[95]

Eddy walked the fine line between needing to assert a public identity as a "reverend" and the overexposure of her as a healing presence that would lead to further censure. Her correspondence became testy when Farlow wrote dutifully: "In response to your suggestion not to be too radical on the subject of protecting you against interviews, I am enclosing herewith a request from the *Philadelphia North American*. . . . It is the leading paper of Philadelphia, and is disposed to be fair. However, I have about made up my mind that we cannot depend upon any newspaper. They will be all right one day and then do the most unheard-of things the next day. . . . The *Philadelphia North American* syndicates all important items, and has among its subscribers many of the leading papers of the West and Middle States. . . . If the *North American* should obtain this article it would appear on the same date in a number of papers which have subscribed for it and which have been previously furnished with a plate ready for the press." Mrs. Eddy replied, "Keep your promise to me once in your life. If you send me or consent to another call for a newspaper article it shall be dealt with by MY CHURCH as AN OFFENCE. NO EXCEPTION unless I request you to do otherwise."[96]

Nonetheless, the media's appetite for news of the religion was difficult if not impossible to control. With the international infrastructure of publications and churches, and Mrs. Eddy's lecture tours that were celebrated for their many healings, the *Boston Globe*'s headlines in the Sunday edition on April 8, 1906, blared, "CHINA NOT READY FOR CHRISTIAN SCIENCE," and reprinted a letter from Eddy intended only for her congregation, published in the house organ, the *Christian Science Journal*, about the "success of CS in benighted China": "Introducing CS into a heathen nation gives it quite another aspect. . . . If the dowager empress could hold her nation, there would be no danger in teaching CS in her country. A war on religion in China would be more fatal than the Boxers' rebellion. Silent prayer in and for a heathen nation is just what is needed. But to teach and to demonstrate Christian Science before the minds of the people are prepared for it, and when the laws are against it, is fraught with danger." Once a Boston newspaper printed an unflattering description, and Farlow wrote to Eddy, "I secured the publication of a correction. . . . A dog seldom receives the rough talk they gave me."[97]

Farlow's work extended to lobbying and monitoring legislation on issues that involved religion and medicine, especially where parents felt the government did not have the "right to tell" them "what healing system he must employ for his child." Finally, Farlow urged church members to become politically active, "making friends with our neighbors who are in the legislating business."[98] In one instance of lobbying in Eddy's home state, New Hampshire, he informed her:

> One thing is certain, the four or five hundred copies which I sent out to the state committees together with their duplicates of the same will reach all the editors in the United States and Canada, and they will get the benefit of it if none of them publish it and undoubtedly it will plant in their consciousness the ideas which it is calculated to convey. . . . If I had had a goodly report of this in the first instance I could have had it in all the Boston papers and could have telegraphed it to some of the larger cities such as New York, Philadelphia, Chicago, Baltimore.[99]

Between 1906 and 1908, *McClure's Magazine* published a hostile series of articles about Eddy, ghostwritten by Willa Cather, not yet a well-known novelist, and bylined by Georgine Milmine; the article, as fictionalized biography, went beyond muckraking, featuring a portrait that was not Eddy.[100]

It was not only her own personal mistakes but also the series of celebrated lawsuits associated with Christian Science that attracted critics, curmudgeons, and muckrakers. For instance, see the Abby Corner case, "the Woodbury" case where a disciple claimed to have become impregnated through mental suggestion, and the "Next Friends" case of 1907, which challenged her mental competency to handle her own financial affairs, the *McClure's* article, and Mark Twain's satire on "Eddypuss" for *Cosmopolitan* magazine. Other publications drew on the *McClure's* articles to disseminate an unflattering image. All this contributed to her progressive withdrawal from public life, along with her advancing age, to the point where newspapers charged she was ill or dead, another charge she had to take on by permitting reporters to interview her in her retirement, according to several recent biographies.

Mrs. Eddy must have been fed up with the mainstream press by this time. In characteristic fashion, she decided to fight fire with fire, after she won the lawsuit challenging her mental competency. She asked her followers to provide an idea of how much it might cost to begin a daily newspaper, the *Christian Science Monitor*, that "would print the truth."[101] The Christian Science Publishing Society responded, and her secretary Adam Dickey replied on August 14, 1908. According to historians, Rev. Eddy was surprised at how expensive the enterprise of starting a national newspaper would become. So she scaled down her idea, describing something that looked very much like the first number of the first issue of the *Christian Journal*, an eight-page tabloid with a projected circulation, "of about fifty or sixty thousand copies, at a much less outlay than the amount stated in your letter. Her intention was not to branch out at once into metropolitan greatness, but rather to begin in a comparatively small way and grow into bigger things with the progress of time. . . . Go ahead with wisdom and economy as your guide."[102]

Presses cost $40,000, and an eight-point font was selected by Eddy herself. By September 15, 1908, she had an eight-page sample prepared, and on November 19, a three-day trial run was printed, with the first real issue appearing on November 25. So many were the advertisements "through the vigorous effort of the advertising department the paper counted in at 12 pages, with 19 columns of that, advertising."[103] The front page included a story about a tariff revision battle in the House Ways and Means Committee, a story about the U.S. armaments budget, and a photo showing progress of the Charles River Dam, which created the Charles River basin in Boston.[104] Though the purpose of the paper was to "be a real newspaper," there was "no intention to camouflage how important Christian Science is to the *Monitor*."[105]

FAITH HEALING

According to historical records of the church, the growth in Mrs. Eddy's popularity resulted from the number of "healings" that took place as a result of her lectures. Church historians attribute the growth of the church and Mrs. Eddy's ability to draw a crowd to "the numbers of healings taking place." From scant audiences at first (ca. 1870s), they grew until it was difficult to get a seat in the 1880s, and advertisements for the lectures carried the warning "come early to get seats." Seats were free, except those in front, which cost fifty cents.[106]

Her trip to Chicago in June 1888 seemed to represent an example of her preaching style at its height.[107] Crowds lined the sidewalks before the doors were opened, and Mrs. Eddy was on the program without her knowing it beforehand. Because the annual meeting of the association had been held the day before, there were still one hundred of her former students in town, along with the delegates. Four thousand visitors were crowded into the hall along with "prominent Chicagoans," and a full table of reporters sat in front of the stage.

A hymn was sung. Mrs. Eddy had by now spoken "on her subject" about four hundred times. The hymn ended, the audience sat down; Mrs. Eddy read the ninety-first Psalm, then spoke for an hour extemporaneously. According to Laura Sargent, a student who related the story later in church records, "the audience was spellbound," it "thrilled" every listener, "there were tears," and all seemed "inspired." When the speech ended, according to the *Chicago Daily Tribune* for June 15, 1888, the audience "arose enmasse and made a rush for the platform . . . mounted the reporters' table and vaulted to the rostrum like acrobats." For more than an hour, old friends, former students, and new admirers surrounded the speaker. The rumor was that eleven healings occurred in the audience that day.[108]

Farlow described her platform style as clear, witty, and succinct with words well chosen. She had an illuminating presence, based on the photographs of her at the time. She was thin, with deep-set, luminous eyes and a halo of white hair, "though looking so peaceful she seemed considerably younger than her years."[109]

Her healing power, as she explained in sermons and in her published writing, was based on the Bible that "teaches us how to heal the sick," and on the healing power of Jesus.

> The entity or ego of man is Spirit and man is but the idea of himself and himself is God of which man is the reflex shadow. . . . Man is the image and likeness of God and should have no other mind but the divine Mind to govern and control this image and likeness of manifestation of God. . . . I mean that man is one of the pictures of God's mind and this picture is a product and not a producer. . . . It is an image and reflection of Intelligence . . . and not a separate mind from God.[110]

Fear was as bad a spiritual influence as disease in Eddy's lexicon; it was a kind of sickness. She cited as illustration the instance of a woman in Lynn, Massachusetts, whose physicians insisted she have ether prior to an operation. After the woman died during the operation from the ether, her sister testified during the trial against the physicians that she had been afraid of the ether, protested against inhaling it, and told the doctors it would kill her. "The evidence was found to be conclusive, and a verdict was returned that death was occasioned, not by the ether, but by fear of inhaling it." Fear was the enemy of belief. The "healing effect followed" belief in Christ, Eddy wrote, leading to understanding the spirit of Christ "which governed" also his human body. This understanding required no clergy, in her view.[111]

Though women at times accounted for four-fifths, two-thirds, or three-quarters of the total membership enrolled, Eddy wanted a religion that included both men and women equally. Her press secretaries and many of the managerial Committee on Publications that spoke through the media about the new religion were men. When Elizabeth Cady Stanton published her *Women's Bible*, Eddy said men and women already had one: "The man's Bible is the woman's [sic] Bible. We cannot have two if the sexes are equal and would not if we could separate the interests of Soul and body from their fraternity in both and give to either prominence of perfectibility."[112]

Given the state of women's health and options for medical care, though, the popular appeal of a religion where women as well as men could study anatomy—and through education gain a measure of medical and spiritual autonomy and possibly authority—would have attracted women. In 1895, Eddy wrote an editorial in the *New Century* heralding "the new woman . . . the equality of men and women," "side by side," "equal partners in all that is worth living for, shall stand the new man with the new woman."[113]

The alternative medical approach to healing and to thinking about self-care appealed to many Americans because it went beyond "Blessed Assurance." It promised religious effectiveness and offered scientific proof. "One case healed is more than other denominations can do," wrote one student to Mrs. Eddy, "whereas all sects can preach and teach more scholarly than the majority of Christian Scientists."[114] "Unless there is less teaching, less church making, and better healing, and more of it—our denomination will sink into the slough of past sects in having a religion of the letter without the Spirit—of doctrine without demonstration."[115] "The early Christians dropped doing the works of Jesus and ran into theorizing and explaining his words. So also Christian Science will be lost to the world if we cease to do the healing works, and others theorize about it—teaching and preaching instead of demonstrating its healing power."[116]

Today, journalists have written in the mainstream and tabloid press countless articles about scientology, an emerging religion often confused with Christian Science because the word "science" is in the title, but the two religions have little in common theologically, beyond the word "science" in the name, and that both were chosen by celebrities in Hollywood in their heyday. The public knows more than they need to about Tom Cruise's ideas on postpartum depression and antidepressants, or about John Travolta's beliefs, but through the midpoint of the twentieth century, Christian Science was the religion of the Hollywood stars.

From the early days of the film industry, the First Church of Pasadena was among the largest in the region. Among those who later had stars on the Boulevard, followers included Joan Crawford, Mary Pickford, Jean Harlow, Mickey Rooney, Gene Autry, Frank Capra, Howard Hawks, Horton Foote, Ginger Rogers, Marilyn Monroe, Audrey Hepburn, Doris Day, Milton Berle, and Henry Fonda, a list that does not indicate their degree of religiosity. Between 1905 and 1907, on the Pacific Coast, as far north as Oregon and Seattle, the Christian Science religion flourished. One celebrated woman healer in Pasadena and Los Angeles at the turn of the century studied medicine for a year at Johns Hopkins, fell ill, and was cured by Edward A. Kimball (1845–1909) in Chicago; she returned to Southern California to be a practitioner. The First Church of Christ in Pasadena added 1,200 members in its first twelve years (1898–1910) and seventy practitioners by 1945. In Los Angeles, five practitioners in 1895 burgeoned to 558 by 1945, adding thirty-seven branch churches.[117]

In 1906, of the estimated 71,000 to 85,000 Christian Scientists in the United States, 4,268 were on the Pacific Coast: 2,753 in California, 591 in Oregon, and 924 in Washington. California had "one of the highest percentages of adherents relative to population in the nation." By 1915, the numbers of Christian Scientists on the Pacific Coast reached 14,000, reflecting a demographic that began among the affluent classes but also included immigrants and working-class people.[118] In part, this was a response to the state of American health care at the turn of the century. It also was in response to what historians suggest motivated many to go to the West; one-third of those who went West were health-seekers pursuing alternative or complementary medical cures.[119]

Mary Baker Eddy was a practical dreamer whose impractical ideas about the power of belief in healing have today been embraced in some areas of alternative medicine. Though the word "placebo" certainly was not in Eddy's vernacular, the phrase epitomizes the theological and medical problem of "mind over matter." Eddy found cause to doubt the value of material medicine, what she called "Matter," and to advocate for the power of the mind to heal the body, preaching the power of the spirit that informs the mind, as one of the keys to understanding health. The placebo effect is the threshold perception in modern mind-body medicine. The respect for the role of belief in healing patients has extended to medical research and clinical practice at today's leading medical schools, including Duke, University of Massachusetts–Amherst, Johns Hopkins, Georgetown, and twenty other schools, Harvard among them. Today in the United States, there are centers conducting research relevant to mind-body medicine in nearly thirty medical schools in the United States, funded by the Templeton and Rockefeller foundations, among other well-respected institutions. Books and magazines have claimed for the Science of Mind a position of leadership in the development of twenty-first-century medicine, as the next chapter discusses.

The language and religious imagination reflected in Christian Science intersects with American literary history, in New England Transcendentalism. Yet the transcendent in Christian Science is very different from transcendentalism, as Robert Peel observed: "A great gulf divides Christian Science from all forms of Transcendentalism. It occurs at the point where Mrs. Eddy's teaching departs entirely from Emersonian 'common sense,' the point at which it denies all reality to matter." Peel concluded that Alcott and the transcendentalists were "halfway between" Emerson and Mrs. Eddy. She went to Emerson to try to heal him during the last months of his life, and described the encounter: "He was as far from accepting Christian Science as a man can be who is a strict moralist. Bronson Alcott is far in advance of him."[120] Eddy knew little about the Hindu and Buddhist traditions, and she seemed to fear them as uncomfortably close to the mesmerists. On her behalf, her secretary Calvin Frye wrote to Septimus Hanna (1844–1921), including a newsclip from a Minnesota paper, "which shows the error is trying hard again to make people believe CS and Buddhism are one & the same thing." He encouraged Hanna to reprint an editorial about a "Hindoo woman" that appeared in the weekly.[121]

Rev. Eddy once wrote to a Rev. F. N. Riale, clarifying the ways in which Christian Science interpreted theological issues about Mind in a way distinct from Buddhism. "Think not," she told him, "that Christian Science tends toward Buddhism or any other 'ism,'" because the study of her religion "destroys such tendencies," to the mystical. She declared that "The doctrine of Buddha, which rests on a heathen basis for Nirvana, represents not the divinity of Christian Science, in which

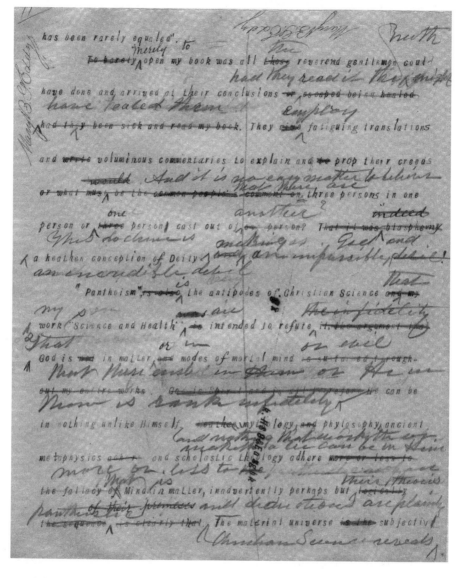

Figure 2.5: Defense of Christian Science. *Typewritten partial draft by Calvin Frye, with autograph emendations in the hand of Rev. Eddy, ca. 1885. Courtesy of MBE Collection.*

Truth, or Christ, finds its paradise in Spirit, in the consciousness of heaven within us—health, harmony, holiness, entirely apart from limitations, which would dwarf individuality in personality and couple evil with good." Christian Science differed in its interpretation of Divine Mind from mystical traditions, she wrote, because in her religion "man is not absorbed in the divine nature, but is absolved by it."[122]

Rev. Eddy's achievements as a leader were remarkable on many counts, and in her resistance to the limits of the cultural imagination that medicine and religion imposed on women, she articulated many of the ideas current in twenty-first-century mind-body and complementary and alternative medicine.

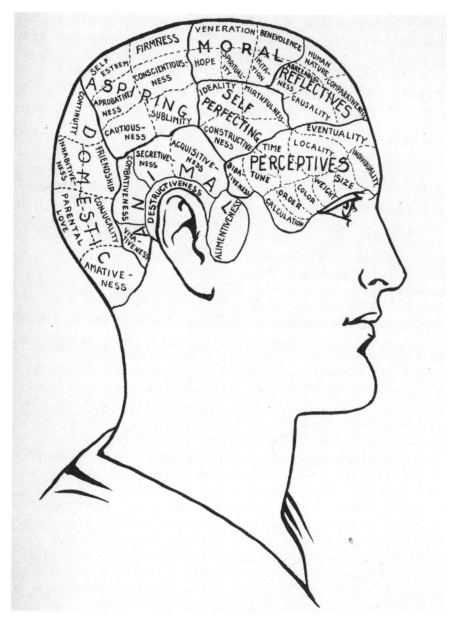

Figure 3.1: A Phrenology Chart of Human Destiny, *by William S. Sadler. From the 1927 edition of his book,* The Physiology of Faith and Fear *(Chicago: A. C. McClurg, 1912). Courtesy of the Newberry Library, Wing Collection Foundation.*

Chapter 3

MEASURING PRAYER
SCIENTIFIC MODELS OF RELIGION

Minds cannot understand, nor systems imitate
The scope of such simplicity

—Thomas Merton

Though the role of prayer in healing is no less controversial today than it was in the late Victorian era of Twain, Eddy, Pulitzer, and William James, the growing popularity today of mind-body medicine, a branch of complementary and alternative health, has drawn renewed attention to the role of faith in healing. There are two schools of research about this; one pertains to curing illness, the other to preventing it. This chapter describes one strand of contemporary discussions and debates about the healing power of prayer in clinical settings—a thread of discourse in a large body of knowledge that combines neurology, psychology, psychiatry, behavioral medicine, Buddhism, and contemplative prayer as factors that can influence healing and sustain health. While the epoch that distinguished the rise of mental science as a basis for new religions about the power of the mind over the body shaped the lives of people during the Eddy era, as the previous chapter described, comparable but very different megatrends shape how we think about prayer and healing in the modern and postmodern American culture, and yet, as this chapter discusses, many comparable ideas are being tried and tested. Today the rise of integrated medicine and the search for a healing presence in clinical trials occurs simultaneously with the growth of global fundamentalism, the emergence of partisan political power among evangelicals, and the boom in fact-filled religious fiction with scriptural lessons, in popular books with transnational markets, and in branded multimedia products that communicate spiritual messages, including those written by celebrity doctors and by gurus from Oprah to Deepak Chopra. While practicing physicians today could not possibly escape the surfeit of media reports about religion and medicine, they are "generally unprepared" to talk with patients about religion, and patients are as slow to bring up the topic with doctors as they would be to ask for medical advice from religious leaders.[1]

Yet the medical research over the past several decades that has attempted to measure the effectiveness of prayer in healing through clinical trials in hospitals, with patients who are ill, is an untold story of a search as bold as it is inconclusive. The scientists who have undertaken research in clinical trials about mind-body medicine and prayer have had to stand up to critics and to the medical establishment, which, understandably, has opposed such unscientific approaches to healing. Because of these investigations over the past three decades, religion courses within the medical curriculum are no longer rare, and medical schools at Duke, Harvard, Johns Hopkins, and Case Western Reserve have developed innovative approaches to "integrated" medicine, an outgrowth of contested "complementary or alternative" practices. Integrated medicine acknowledges nonmedical factors, including nutrition, emotion, and sustainable environments, and recognizes that prayer, meditation, altruism, optimism, and forgiveness have a role in healing. What is most remarkable about this development in the history of American religion and medicine is not that research scientists who are published in peer-reviewed medical journals have "concluded" so little, but that they continue to investigate the mystery of a possible avenue of healing beyond the rational realm—and attempt to explain it physiologically, framing it scientifically with exact protocols that measure religiousness.

Part of what drives this current megatrend in integrated medicine is the consumer-driven realization of the failures of traditional or regular medicine, such as the recalls of toxic pharmaceutical prescriptions that routinely fill the headlines. This expression of a need to find an alternative to prescription cures can be understood within the context of historical place in American culture for "prescribing," the heroic cures and precarious situation of women's health in the nineteenth century, popular medical advice books, the era of fads and quackery that led to the development of Mind Cure and New Thought movements, and medically resistant religions such as Christian Science, among other sects such as Seventh-Day Adventists and Jehovah's Witnesses. Such religions flourished because many people feared both the unreliability and the power of American medicine. The history of American medicine is one in which the rise of faith-based healing practices occurred simultaneously with other significant trends in the interpretation of scripture; in that respect, the early twenty-first century resembles the earlier turn-of-the-twentieth-century era.

Deep ambivalence marks the dialogue among physicians in response to "advances" about using prayer as an intervention in medicine: "Medicine and prayer don't mix," according to Sloan, one representative voice among many other doctors objecting with no uncertainty about controversial approaches to faith and wellness that incorporate prayer or meditative practices in clinical settings. Sloan wrote that including religion in the practice of medicine is "simply unacceptable," because it decreases the time doctors have to spend with patients talking about real disease; may "cause harm," by coercing patients; crosses ethical boundaries; and is "bad for religion": "Bringing religion into the laboratory subjects it to the reductionism of scientific materialism, stripping away all elements of transcendence. The recent report that religious experience is based on the neurochemistry of the serotonin system in the brain is a perfect example of how religion is trivialized by studying it scientifically."[2]

Though many doctors undoubtedly will continue to object to the continuing research that investigates religion and medicine, if belief in the power of prayer to heal is a significant variable in health, along with psychosocial and behavioral factors, then science has a real need to be able to measure effectiveness of religion as a medical intervention. Many scientists argue that the inconclusiveness of studies to date results from poor design, and there have been a number of attempts to provide the appropriate research protocols through which to study the effect of religion in medicine.

The idea of trying to test for effectiveness of religiousness as a buffer against disease has created new research models, ethical issues about informed consent for researchers, and an emerging body of literature in interdisciplinary fields, such as neurotheology, psychoneuroimmunology, and psychoendocrinology. Scientific studies have demonstrated that religion can be a buffer against the disease-causing biochemical reactions of a mind under stress, and can reduce the physiological impact of emotions. Scientists and doctors long have questioned why some people remain healthy and others do not, even though both may live in equally stressful environments. Some people's negative thoughts put them into states as stressful as reality. Anxiety, fears, or phobias are the toxic emotional states that take their toll on the heart. Many physician researchers are interested in all modes of faith practices that can buffer stress, including religion, social networks, and other lifestyle factors, including psychological factors such as the ability to think positively about negative situations.[3]

The focus in this chapter is on the emerging narrative about what scientific protocols, effective methods, and reliable instruments devised to measure prayer as a therapeutic intervention through clinical trials in research have been published in the medical literature. The discussion is based on an environmental scan and content analysis of the body of literature in medical journals published recently and accessible through the National Library of Medicine. This is a representative rather than comprehensive survey, because the literature is simply too extensive for this small volume. Jonas and Crawford counted 1,200 references in English alone and 200 controlled clinical studies six years ago, and since then, the research stream has increased: "None were about placebo effects and all were trying to prove that healing exists."[4] Of the recent 850 studies, random samples consisted of those people who went to church and prayed, and who had strong social networks, with healthful lifestyles that "contributed to their overall health," so it was difficult to separate their prayer habits or religious beliefs from other behavioral factors.[5] Among the elderly cohort, rates of depression and anxiety tended to decrease among those professing some religious beliefs, but

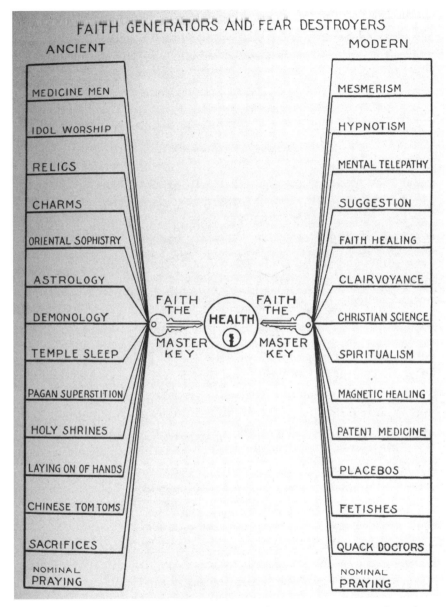

Figure 3.2: Diagram showing factors influencing ancient and modern creation and destruction of faith. Faith Generators and Fear Destroyers, *by William S. Sadler. From his book,* The Physiology of Faith and Fear *(Chicago: A. C. McClurg, 1912). Courtesy of the Newberry Library, Wing Collection Foundation.*

the problem for scientists is how to measure the gradations of religiousness, how to separate those who rely on religion because of the utility of the social structure of churches, from those whose deepest intuitive faith relies on interpretations such as submission to God's will. Not all studies correlated the observation of religious practices and social support, considered a key health factor by many researchers. Nor did all studies find that more church attendance contributed to longevity, though some have.[6] Krause found that among the elderly worried by financial strain, those who gave support *to others* rather than received support *from* their congregation experienced a more positive health benefit, but this conclusion is tempered by the unknown variables, since those needing the support may have been in a more frail condition.[7] Doctors are trying to understand more fully how religion buffers the effects of stress on the brain; "although research in this area is just beginning, there is evidence to suggest that the adoption of stress-buffering beliefs and behaviors will have a beneficial effect on health," according to research scientists.[8]

PRAYER AS THERAPEUTIC

The Centers for Disease Control (CDC) found in its most recent and largest survey, of 31,000 Americans, that prayer was the least common therapeutic intervention in 1990; twelve years later, it was the most common.[9] A large percentage of those who said they used mind-body medicine as their "preferred" approach to healing are praying for themselves for a specific medical concern, for others who are ill, or in healing rituals or prayer groups. Evidence cited by Harvard summarized the prayer patterns as applied to specific diseases. For improved health generally, as well as critical illness, cancer, arthritis, burns, birth complications, blood pressure, and addictions, "numerous studies" have been conducted, but in each case, the need for "further" research is declared "before conclusions can be drawn."[10] Another recently published national survey reported that 75 percent of Americans prayed for wellness in 1998; 22 percent for specific conditions. Of those praying for specific conditions, 69 percent felt that prayer helped. Of the three-quarters of Americans who prayed for wellness in 1998, "with or without specific conditions, only 11 percent of those felt free to talk about it with their physicians."[11] Patient apprehension of doctors and the time constraints under which most physicians work inhibit communication between patient and provider so that a chasm exists between what should be and what could be in communication about health in a clinical or therapeutic setting.

Prayer is one therapy within mind-body medicine, part of the broad category of integrative medicine defined by the National Center for Complementary and Alternative Medicine at the National Institutes of Health (NCCAM), which predicts that "Integrative medicine will be seen as providing novel insights and tools for human health, practiced by health-care providers skilled and knowledgeable in the multiple traditions and disciplines that contribute to the healing arts."[12] Some doctors resist the religiously pluralistic approaches to healing implied by these categories as defined at the highest levels of the National Institutes of Health, even if used "together with" conventional medicine, because "alternative" medicine subordinates medical knowledge to folk or religious knowledge. Most see mind-body medicine as "complementary" to regular medicine, rather than "alternative" according to a recent survey.[13]

The idea that certain people "exude a healing presence" is not idiosyncratic to late nineteenth-century American culture, nor a demonstration of a naïve strain in the postmodern American culture. As a physician-researcher observed recently, belief in a healing presence is widely shared across all cultures. Suffering is endemic to the human condition, and though various religions have interpreted the role of suffering in spiritual growth differently, over the ages beliefs in healing through plants, people, prayer, and other sacred rituals changed and is changing, shaped by popular ideas, subcultures, and notions of cultural identity. Science has spent "less time than it should have" looking into the cultural nuance of belief in medicine; scientific investigations into the "mechanism" of prayer in healing have fallen short because scientists investigating belief have asked the wrong questions, according to Jonas and Crawford.[14]

The scientific investigation of prayer as a therapeutic intervention in healing differs from prescribing meditation in mind-body medicine to reduce stress and relax the cardiovascular system, creating conditions conducive to wellness. The first is seeking a cure; the second is about maintaining a state of calm emotion and a quiet mind that contribute to longevity. Scientists today are testing prayer as a healing intervention

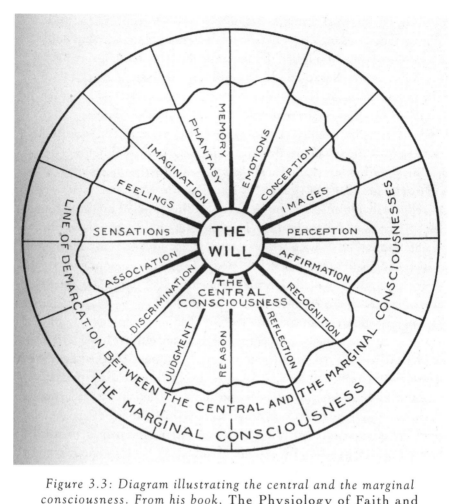

Figure 3.3: Diagram illustrating the central and the marginal consciousness. From his book, The Physiology of Faith and Fear *(Chicago: A. C. McClurg, 1912). Courtesy of the Newberry Library, Wing Collection Foundation.*

among patients in a diseased state. But prayer is considered only one among many equal modes of healing in the contemporary American climate of medical pluralism, including practices from Eastern medical traditions such as qui gong and the "laying on of hands" in therapeutic touch.

The National Institutes of Health estimates that the number of visits to complementary medical care providers currently exceeds the number of visits to primary care physicians, a trend that has strengthened since

NIH's first survey in 1990. Sixty-two percent of the 31,000 Americans surveyed in 2002 reported having used prayer as a Complementary and Alternative Medicine (CAM) therapy within the past year; prayer was among twenty other alternative practices listed as options, including meditation, yoga, reiki, tai chi, diet, megavitamins, chiropractic, massage, biofeedback, energy healing, folk medicine, guided imagery, herbs and homeopathic treatment, hypnosis, progressive relaxation, qui gong, and deep breathing.[15] Most people who used CAM and who did not use prayer as part of mind-body medicine preferred "biological approaches."[16]

BOTANICAL AND BIOLOGICAL CURES

The National Institutes of Health, NCCAM division, funded by Congress, links interdisciplinary concepts about wellness: scientific, religious, and folk approaches to medicine. NCCAM reports that alternative and complementary practices, "once considered unorthodox in the United States can become part of the mainstream health-care repertoire following demonstrations of safety and efficacy by rigorous scientific investigation." For example, those practices include

> acupuncture . . . prescribed to manage pain and sometimes to control nausea associated with chemotherapy . . . and to treat cocaine addiction. Among the first drugs for treatment of high blood pressure was reserpine from the herb Rauwolfia sepentina, described many centuries ago in Indian Ayruvedic monographs. Indeed, some our most important drugs . . . are derivatives of the active ingredients identified in herbal remedies. Such drugs of botanical origin include digitalis for the treatment of congestive heart failure and vincristine, and more recently taxol, for treatment of cancers. . . . Other herbal remedies and CAM practices may prove effective in preventing and treating chronic diseases, possibly reducing the costs of health-care, as well as advancing our understanding of how healing works.[17]

Alternative modes of healing are not without risks. Dr. Herbert Benson of Harvard Medical School, among the early and leading advocates for the power of belief in wellness and mind-body medicine, expressed caution about some aspects of CAM. He observed that while "medicine needs to change to empower patients and take advantage of patients' faith and beliefs," there is no "wisdom" in substituting "one set of drugs and procedures for another set of drugs and procedures." The most "natural" form of healing is that which the patient does for him or herself," he wrote. From the patients' perspective, complementary and alternative medical approaches "have a great appeal," both in conjunction with conventional medicine and also as an alternative to a health care system that has left them frustrated, as Benson put it when describing the public confidence level.[18]

More recently, Dr. Jerome Groopman of Harvard Medical School advocated in a *Wall Street Journal* editorial that recent findings in a study sponsored by NCCAM of 1,583 patients given glucosamine and chondroitin sulfate proved "ineffective" for curing osteoarthrisis, and another trial about the ineffective herb saw palmetto for symptoms of enlarged prostate glands "should mark a sea change in how the public views such treatments." In the osteoarthritis study, 60 percent of patients receiving the placebo (plus Celebrex) reported significant improvement. "A good doctor distills magic from medicine," Groopman wrote, as he went about trying to reverse the public image of "natural" medication as benign.[19]

The fact of the matter is that nature is full of toxins and poisons, but we are too far removed from the Walter Channing and Sophia Peabody era to remember collectively that once in American culture there was an era when ideas about regular medicine included heroic cures, some of them prescribing natural substances in toxic formulations. Today such toxins routinely save the lives of cancer patients, despite the brutal side effects. "Chemotherapy drugs vincristine and taxol, are derived, respectively, from the periwinkle plant and the Pacific yew tree," Groopman explained.[20] However, he wrote, the public needs to be wary about many faddish herbal supplements and megavitamins, and people need to be especially cautious when mixing the natural and the pharmaceutical, a lethal combination caused by lack of disclosure by the patient and ignorance on the part of the physician. For example, St. John's Wort proved to interfere with anti-HIV protease drugs; Compound Q extracted from the Chinese cucumber widely used in Asia as an abortifacient caused severe toxic reactions among patients, inducing coma; and laetrile extracted from apricot pits touted as a cancer cure caused people to reject standard chemotherapy drugs. Shark cartilage that was supposed to cause tumors to recede but failed to do so is another faddish cancer cure in alternative medicine that has not succeeded, amid much publicity. Herbal supplements found today in any run-of-the-mill health food store are dangerous when mixed with prescription medicine, or certain substances are dangerous alone, such as ephedra, which U.S. Health and Human Services banned in 2003.

The controversial difference between those relying on natural versus prescribed medications constitutes "a considerable risk," according to the government.[21] Yet the negative outcomes of natural cures are offset by the many new pharmaceutical products that also fail to heal, Groopman observed in what is a classic understatement. The NIH division that supported and fosters the legitimacy of alternative cures, NCCAM, is supported by taxpayers and was created by Congress, which offers a type of legitimacy in the public eye. Yet "despite the scientific evidence to the contrary, many believers keep the faith about the power of alternative medicine to heal," Groopman wrote. Finally, he predicted that "as science spreads" its evidence about the ineffectiveness of herbal supplements and cures, the "faithful will fall away," and the numbers of believers will "shrink," he predicted.[22]

The current climate, though, suggests the trend is not in that direction. Patients push for an integrated approach that incorporates leeway for natural cures. Rather than rejecting these ideas, physicians need to know about the adverse side effects of combining pharmaceutical drugs and herbal supplements that "regular" doctors like Groopman would appear to resist and to realize that many patients do not tell their doctor the whole story. Agdal argues the case for practicing physicians today having a greater understanding about medical practices that include methods rooted in ethnicity and religion.[23]

ETHNIC APPROACHES TO HEALING

Sternberg posed the crucial question for the emerging age of scientific medical pluralism, healing through both conventional medicine and complementary approaches such as mind-body medicine, in which meditation and also prayer play a therapeutic role: "If the belief in the power of a drug to cure gives it at least a third of its ability to heal, why shouldn't prayer and fervent belief alone be an effective cure that works in part through those same nerve pathways and hormones that traduce the placebo effect?" Only science can provide evidence about what happens within patients physiologically as they pray, but rather than get involved in what Sternberg calls the effort to "refute" or "support" its power, she concluded that the "nerve pathways and molecules that effect immune cell function activated by belief in a pill can also be activated by prayer."[24]

Koenig cited "at least sixty studies" that measured diminishment of pain and better "coping" through religious beliefs among patients with serious medical conditions such as arthritis, diabetes, kidney disease, cancer, heart disease, AIDS, sickle cell, and ALS. He related the story of one elderly patient whose religious ways of coping brought about a reduction in pain, to illustrate what happens physiologically when anxious patients pray. They become less anxious about what they cannot control, and their tense muscles relax. He used a clinical case history of one individual to help illustrate how prayer helps a patient "stop obsessing and turn things over to God," reducing the anxiety many patients feel about being ill, and their feelings of helplessness and lack of control. Koenig's view supported Sternberg's description of the neural and hormonal pathways that are influenced by prayer: "Religious beliefs and practices like prayer could influence physical as well as mental sympathetic and parasympathetic nerve tracks that connect thoughts and emotions in the brain to the circulatory system. . . . If religious beliefs and prayer help patients cope better with illness . . . then they may counteract stress-related physiological" systems that "impair healing."[25]

Many ethnic traditions value the folk medicine that blends myth and habit, belief and superstition as part of an inherited cultural identity. Recent research by Hsiao supports the hypothesis that traditional and folk medicine among ethnic groups "results in a pattern of CAM use that varies" according to demographics. In Hsiao's view, the pattern of use is determined by ethnicity. Many CAM therapies that were first folk traditions are classified by the National Center for Complementary and Alternative Medicine as being part of the movement.[26] Embedded in popular thinking about health, both ethnicity and race influence how many people approach the problem of suffering and their hope for the possibility of wellness. Hsiao and his associates argue that physicians need to be aware of the reality of ethnicity and race in their approaches to prescriptions, especially where pharmaceutical or surgical intervention may conflict with folk medicine that patients might not be willing disclose to physicians.

Hsiao found, for example, a pattern of ethnic-specific treatments. Asian Americans use traditional Chinese medicine: acupuncture, green tea, and soy products. American Indians use a Native American healer to cure the sick and participate in healing rituals. African Americans use garlic pills, and a high percentage of them rely on having others pray for them; Latinos use a curandero. Only Caucasians relied on masseurs and osteopaths with any frequency.[27] In Mikhail's earlier study among Hispanics in Los Angeles, the majority preferred conventional medicine to complementary practices—if they could afford it. Suzuki's research among physicians in Japan demonstrates how differently American culture defines CAM from other cultures. Among the most frequent users of the herb-based Kampo with conventional medicine were the Japanese doctors themselves who had been educated in the West.[28]

INTERCESSORY PRAYER

The historical benchmarks in this field are the key studies of intercessory prayer by Byrd in 1988, Harris in 1999, and Benson in 2000 and 2006, though there are also others. These studies have concentrated on the effect of prayer on heart patients in hospitals for bypass surgery and other remedial measures to save their lives. The effort has been and will continue to be no less controversial than it was in the days of Mark Twain and Joseph Pulitzer, when they questioned Rev. Eddy's sanity for trying the same thing.

The 1988 study by Byrd is cited in the literature as the landmark study in our own era about the impact of prayer on health.[29] Byrd patterned his study on an earlier one by Galton in 1872, three years before Eddy founded the religion based on prayer in healing and rejection of medicine.[30] Galton's suggestion at the end of the nineteenth century had been that medical researchers had an option: they could look either at individual cures, central to the many claims of healing during the quack era, or observe demographic cohorts or classes of patients about whom specific conclusions could be drawn about cures. In this regard, Galton was far ahead of other scientists during his day.

Byrd was motivated in 1988 to address the gap between his own era and Galton's work in 1872. Byrd wrote, "Praying for help and healing is a fundamental concept in practically all societies, though the object to which these prayers are directed varies among the religions of the world. . . . However, the medical literature contains no scientific evidence either confirming or negating the healing effectiveness of intercessory prayer."[31] He cited one research article that had been published in the last century in the *Archives of Internal Medicine*, by C. G. Roland titled, "Does Prayer Preserve?" Byrd concluded that he could "presume" the beneficial effects of prayer on patients, based on Roland's research. Byrd wrote, "The medical literature contains no scientific evidence either confirming or negating the healthy effectiveness of intercessory prayer. In only a few studies have scientific methods been used to attempt to determine whether or not prayer is therapeutically effective, and these studies have been inconclusive."[32]

Between 1982 and 1983, Byrd studied the therapeutic effects of intercessory prayer in a San Francisco hospital's coronary care unit, in a prospective randomized double-blind protocol over ten months, with 393 patients total: 192 in the group who would receive prayer and 201 in a control group who would not. He sought to determine if there were any effect on the patients' medical condition and how these effects might be characterized. Byrd found that among those who had been prayed for, patients required less breathing assistance, antibiotics, and diuretics than the patients in the control group. His method included recruiting "born-again" Christians, Roman Catholics, and Protestants to pray for patients, matching the patients with intercessors according to their respective denomination. They were led in daily prayer outside the hospital by a coordinator. Staff and patients knew the study was being conducted and that heart patients were being prayed for, but not in which group patients were clustered. *Patients who objected were dropped from the study.* Those who prayed knew the patient's first name, condition, and diagnosis. They were asked to pray, verbatim, "for a rapid recovery and for prevention of complications and death, in addition to other areas of prayer they believed to be beneficial to patients."[33] His Christocentric approach would be unthinkable in today's

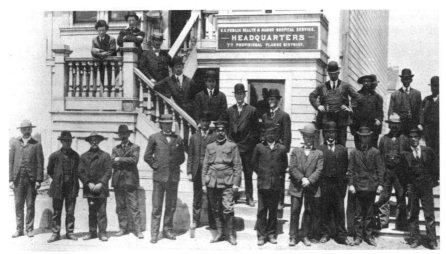

Figure 3.4: G. A. Weyer *(front row, seventh from left, in uniform), acting assistant surgeon general of the U.S. Public Health Department, with twenty-six health workers, San Francisco, California. Photograph, ca. 1907–1909. Courtesy of the National Library of Medicine.*

pluralistic environment. The limitations of Byrd's denominational outlook are cited in today's literature as a weakness of his research design.

Ten years later, Harris reiterated the study, and his findings uphold and are consistent with Byrd's. But when Harris published his results in 1999, public attitudes were different. Because media had raised public awareness of the issues in CAM, because many of the books by physicians had become global best sellers, and because of the widespread popularity of Buddhism and yoga as part of alternative self-care, Harris's results about using prayer as a medical intervention stirred tempers in a dialogue published in the medical literature across the globe.

Harris tested the power of intercessory prayer on 990 patients consecutively admitted to a hospital's coronary care unit and divided into two groups, ones who would be prayed for, and a control group that would not. "The design was a randomized, controlled, double-blind, prospective parallel group trial." None of the 990 patients knew they were being prayed for, and those doing the praying were "a team" who prayed for them daily over four weeks; they did not know the patients, nor anything about their personal history.

Based on slightly lower level of complications among those receiving prayers, Harris concluded that "prayer may be an effective adjunct to standard medical care." The Harris study differed from Byrd's in several ways. There was neither informed consent nor prescreening of patients based on belief. The hospital granted an exemption to Harris, so that patients would not have to sign giving their informed consent to be prayed for, "because it was agreed that there was no known risk associated with receiving remote, intercessory prayer, and no known risk for the patients in the usual care group associated with not receiving extra prayer." Anticipating controversy about informed consent, Harris defended his choice, arguing that the process of getting informed consent might make patients nervous, or in other ways agitate their condition, causing harm. Intercessors were "asked to pray for twenty-eight days regardless of what happened to the patient," though they received "no feedback regarding the patient's progress during this time."

Harris concluded a bit too simply for his critics, writing that "[w]hether this affected their commitment to prayer is unknown." So if prayer was considered a "minimal" risk, what does that say about the confidence of investigators into its positive power to heal? Harris discussed, but did not make any allowance in his research design for what he called "background" prayer, those that patients "would receive anyway," from relatives, coreligionists or friends, with or without the trial. In what Harris clearly seemed to think was an advance in research design over the Byrd study, prayer teams were "any" denomination, screened only by their agreement with the idea of a "personal God who hears and answers prayers made on behalf of the sick." They were organized into fifteen teams of five. Prayers were offered individually, not in groups. Harris wrote that neither his study nor that of Byrd a decade earlier tried to explain why patients seemed to be slightly better off with prayer. "This trial was designed to explore not a mechanism but a phenomenon." Comparing his study to the intuitive work of scientists in the eighteenth century who knew before they could prove it that citrus prevented scurvy, Harris concluded, "Chance still remains a possible explanation of our results." The results were important because of the interest in alternative and complementary medicine "rapidly" growing in the United States, Harris wrote, where prayer "therapy" was becoming accepted "as part of CAM."[34]

The study by Harris provoked considerable comment in the medical literature. Larry Dossey, M.D., an author of several best sellers and a proponent of psychokinesis from his home in New Mexico, a phenomenon that he defined as the "anomalous perturbation of distant events," commented at length. He supported research about therapeutic uses of intercessory prayer because of his interest in psychokinesis; it's "not nonsense," nor is telepathy, Dossey argued from his own "considerable evidence." Dossey observed that not only history but also physics and the history of American science were on his side. Citing a meta-analysis of 832 studies done by sixty-eight investigators, he argued the case for research by those whose "mental efforts" tried to "change biological systems." Among those systems were the recovery rate of animals from anesthesia, wound healing in animals, biochemical reactions in vitro, and the rate at which bacteria reproduced in a petri dish. Dossey cited statistical evidence from another recent survey as demonstrating "nearly 39% of American biologists, physicists and mathematicians said that they believed in God."

Many people think of scientists as skeptics, "a healthy state of things for scientific inquiry," Dossey concluded, warning against a "type of dogmatic materialism" that might exclude the possibility of intercessory prayer to bring about healing. Further, he argued against the protests from conservatives in the medical establishment opposing such studies as not well grounded. Though some argued against the research by Harris and Byrd because they thought it was wrong "in principle," Dossey replied that while they were correct in thinking that science dealt "with facts and not miracles," and the results of Harris's study suggested that "happenings presumably follow natural law and are not considered miraculous," he cited Newton, whose observations about gravity had initially been met by charges from his contemporaries that he had surrendered to mysticism. Newton's situation was similar to "criticism that prayer researchers underwent today," Dossey cautioned, asking his peers to refrain from "calling things miraculous," because "the subsequent course of history may reveal that these terms reflect little more than our own ignorance." Dossey concluded, "Today we are as baffled by the remote effects of prayer as Newton's critics were by the distant effects of gravity. . . . The debate surrounding intercessory prayer may also diminish with time," but medical knowledge about the "mechanism" of intercessory prayer might remain."[35]

From the Netherlands, a physician derided the debate as ludicrous. Willem van der Does provided a mathematical formula for "chance," an explanation that Harris used to account for his results, satirizing his own commentary as his "first transatlantic telepathy work."[36] A physician from Australia, Jennifer Smith, interpreted Harris's results as having within the protocol an inherent bias, since those who had had access to the patient charts were aware of which patients were in which groups, and, after all, if the results had shown no positive effect, "it would have been difficult to publish an article showing that remote intercessory prayer had no effect on clinical outcomes."[37] Prakesh Pande, an Indian doctor practicing in Indianapolis, questioned the whole concept of a randomized study as simply impossible, and failed "to understand" the suggestion that "further randomized studies" were called for. He observed that people had been praying since ancient times, and he quoted the biblical caution that men should "not put God to the test." Arguing that a "pure randomization" for intercessory prayer is not possible, he "failed to see" any reason for further studies about the healing power of prayer.[38]

Sloan and Bagiella agreed that such investigations in prayer should cease. They raised the problems with the method's limitations to the Judeo-Christian tradition and objected to such research because of the "significant ethical issues raised by the conclusion that prayer should be added to the list of medical interventions." They wrote that "religion does not need medical science to validate its rituals," and that to further study prayer "trivializes" religion.[39]

Another physician in Chicago, Julie Goldstein, attacked the method of waiving informed consent for those patients in clinical trials who were already acutely ill, perhaps terminally. As in Byrd's 1988 study, many people, she argued, would be like she had been, initially interested by the idea that a little prayer could do no one any harm. But since then she changed her mind; it could perhaps do harm. The informed consent required for such studies could cause harm to patients, who might be alarmed unduly that death might be imminent, or in other ways become stressed, raising heart rate and blood pressure—in a cardiac unit, at that! She jibed that maybe a god might view such a request unfavorably from a nonbeliever, and observed that doctors who conducted such research were treading into the unknown territory of neurotheology. Finally, she argued, there was the reputation of the hospitals to consider, and the very remote possibility that of the nearly one thousand patients under study, none would not objected to have people whom they did not know praying for them.[40]

A doctor from Minneapolis, Hammerschmidt, thought the ethical problems even worse than the practical ones, and wrote, "One should think long and hard before enrolling an uninformed, nonconsenting patient as a subject in a study that he or she might find blasphemous."[41] Sandweiss, a San Diego physician, called the whole business "pseudo-scientific mischief."[42] Hoover and Margolick thought the findings of efficacy so slight they were insignificant.[43] A doctor from New York, Rosner, questioned why prayer had to be scientifically proven at all since it is well known that "prayer can ameliorate or prevent disease and despondency. Prayer sets a psychological frame of mind to allow the body's psyche to be at rest with itself. Since ancient times, it has been known that the state of mind of a sick person influences the responses to treatment."[44] And ten physicians coauthored, another piece (Galishoff et al.), "Perhaps the irony of the study is that the outcome was the same despite fewer interventions from the prayer group. Perhaps the real conclusion is that God's grace is greater than our skills and immeasurable by our tools. Like many before them, the investigators might have missed the real message of the "study": that despite our arrogance, God's omnipotence is beyond our ability to add or detract."[45]

The worldwide response to Harris's study led to subsequent studies, including two by Benson (2001, 2006) and one by Katterndahl (2004) where there was an attempt to correlate "interpersonal belief in prayer efficacy" as "consistent with the literature showing the relevance of personal belief in health and well-being in general," and recommendations to future researchers in this area that the factor of belief in prayer be accounted for in the research design.[46]

Though "inconclusive" as scientific research, many found the benefits of intercessory prayer "compelling."[47] The psychological profile of those being prayed for as believers, they argued, had been well established. Benson, among others, had established it in his body of work on mind-body research since the 1970s. The researchers argued that "inter-personal factors such as hope, belief, faith, and attitudes can influence health outcomes and that the "role of personal belief"—"belief in the power of prayer," and "belief that a personal problem can be resolved"— is a significant variable modifying the "association between intercessory prayer and a specific personal outcome.[48]

Brian Bolton observed in an editorial that, while eight "carefully conducted clinical trials" had been published in refereed journals with-out any evidence that intercessory prayer had "any measurable bene-fits for the patients," he did not support those who had lambasted the effort.[49] To measure prayer in such experimental studies should not be "shunned" under the guise of thinking God was trivialized in the pro-cess.[50] The search for a healing presence entails a "physiology of belief," which researchers distinguish from religious rituals, such as a "laying on of hands" or other actions that involve physical contact.[51]

The role of healing prayer is complicated theologically as well as sci-entifically. In recent studies, Benson tried to demonstrate the effective-ness of intercessory prayer on the recovery of cardiac bypass patients after surgery.[52] Benson had found that *patients who were prayed for were worse off than those who were not.* According to his staff at Harvard's Mind Body Institute, the second study had been completed three years prior to its release. Understandably, Benson must have been cautious about releas-ing his negative results, which disputed the earlier studies by Byrd and Harris. Before releasing his three-year-old data, the Mind Body Institute at Harvard Medical School (now at Massachusetts General Hospital) employed the global public relations firm Edelmann Worldwide to han-dle the media relations as the results were published in the cardiology literature in 2006. Edelmann scheduled a national conference call among physicians interested in the results with key researchers involved in the study to occur on the day prior to the *Journal's* publication, ostensibly to blunt the anticipated criticism that would follow such results, by full press access between the authors and all interested parties. The confer-ence call was moved up a day when Edelmann found *The New York Times* published a front-page story about the negative results of the study the day before the conference call and scheduled release of the data. Proving inconclusive results or the benign quality of prayer was one thing, but proving deleterious results raised the spectre of informed consent, ethics, and what Leder called the "spooky" side of the entire debate.[53]

In Benson's Study of the therapeutic effects of intercessory prayer (STEP), he and his colleagues tested in 2000 and in 2001 (the latter published in 2006) whether having people pray for someone who is ill would help them recover from illness, a claim "not supported by well-controlled clinical trials." Benson wanted to see if patients who knew they were being prayed for differed in recovery times from those who did not know they were being prayed for. Benson's method was the following: patients undergoing coronary artery bypass graft surgery were randomly divided into three groups of about six hundred patients. The first two groups learned "they may or may not" be prayed for; the first group was prayed for, the second group was not. A third group was prayed for, as they had been promised.

Patients in the trial "were informed that their first names and first initial of their last name might be forwarded to three Christian prayer groups. The prayer groups were Catholic and Protestants. In what would prove to be a controversial fault in method, *Benson noted that his researchers were "unable to locate" other denominations.* Preoperatively, subjects were asked whether they believed in spiritual healing and whether friends, relatives, and/or members of their religious institution would be praying for them. Starting the night before surgery, and for the following two weeks, the intercessory prayers, "beginning at midnight," commenced. The same daily updated list was faxed to each of three intercessory prayer groups every weekday for the duration: the list was posted in a central location not later than 7:15 p.m. EST each evening, with intercessory prayer beginning by midnight for patients on the list. The intercessors agreed to add the phrase, "for a successful surgery with a quick, healthy recovery and no complications" to their usual prayers.

Among the group who knew they were being prayed for, there were more complications (59 percent) than among the other two groups, uncertain about whether or not they were receiving prayers. Significant negative findings resulted from the patients' awareness of being prayed for, which led to a "higher incidence of complications."[54] In the discussion of his findings published in the *American Heart Journal*, Benson concluded that intercessory prayer "had no effect," and knowing someone was praying for them led to a higher rate of complications than among those who were uncertain. Among the possible explanations researchers offered were that perhaps such prayer was ineffective, or that the thirty days after surgery may not be "appropriate or relevant" to the effects of intercessory prayer—and the difference "may also be well because of chance." Though Harris had used "chance" to explain results in a prayer study, Benson's use of the term came under heavier fire.

An editorial in the *American Heart Journal* suggested that the mention of "chance" in a results section was "unscientific" and "unusual."[55] Among the conclusions in the results section were that the flaws in the study might reside with those who were doing the praying and that the research design had given intercessors insufficient connection with the patients for whom they were praying. Though they had "used a standard study intention during their prayers," they had been "informed by FAX rather than by personal association" with the identity of the people for whom they were praying. Benson's researchers did not interfere with "background" prayer, those offered by family and friends, because it would "have been unethical and impractical" to have asked the patients to "alter any plans" for prayer support through their existing network. Benson concluded that at the time of enrollment, all patients were receiving some prayers from family or friends, and so the *"chance"* element in his findings might have been attributable to the "uneven numbers of prayers received from people other than the assigned prayer groups."[56]

The *American Heart Journal* editorial raised larger issues, such as that the study authors missed the forest for the trees: the trial might have "provided insight into the possible role of a placebo effect." Further, the journal's editors charged that Benson had tread on very thin ice ethically, and that his assumptions about prayer were culturally embedded and reflected bias rather than scientific objectivity. Benson's conclusion that prayer was "only capable of doing good, if it does anything at all," and that negative effects of prayer were relegated to voodoo or negative thoughts, reflected a cultural bias, editors claimed. Yet the "cultural dichotomy is medically problematic and ethically unacceptable in the setting of a clinical trial performing structured experimentation on human subjects," editors argued. Though researchers were as scientifically exact in their design structure as possible, the "question of safety in the final data interpretation promotes a dangerously ambiguous message to investigators who might be inclined to do research in this area in the future."[57] Finally, the editors pointed out, fear in scientific and religious contexts is a significant variable that can alter results in mind-body medicine. It would seem reasonable to conclude that the patients who knew that they were being prayed for associated prayer with impending death, creating complications.[58]

The idea of distance in the intercessory prayer trials interested some scientists far more than the religious dimensions of the question, or the ethical issues, the rigor, or the question of authenticity of belief. Two studies are noteworthy. One delved directly into the idea of "distant healing" using quantum mechanics, energy transmission, and "warps" in time-space.

"Physics-based models . . . are suggestive" in exploring the "disjunctions and compatibilities between modern physics and . . . distant healing," the author of the study wrote. "Perhaps people, like particles, can become entangled so they behave as one system with instantaneous and unmediated correlations across a distance," she suggested. Perhaps, she continued, conscious healing intention could act like quantum mechanics, which "collapses a probabilistic wave function into a single outcome," and that "[p]erhaps conscious healing intention can act similarly, helping to actualize one of a series of possibilities: for example, recovery from a lethal tumor."

The concept of "distant intentionality" led researchers into a second study to construct an experiment using eleven native Hawaiian healers with more than two decades experience. Achterberg and her coauthors attempted to fit a scientific paradigm containing historic concepts from the late nineteenth century, ideas such as electrical magnetism or "energy healing" and the ability to heal others at a distance, into the same concept model as "efficacy of prayer."[59] Researchers used the term "distant intentionality" as the umbrella concept that "subsumes" prayer, energy healing, healing at a distance, spiritual healing, therapeutic touch, transpersonal imagery, and remote mental healing. The authors cited a comprehensive literature review published by Jonas and Crawford that concluded "there is a growing interest in the scientific community" about the distant intentionality approach to healing, and that twenty-two hundred published reports on "spiritual healing, prayer, energy medicine, and mental intention effects" had been included.[60] Rather than trying to prove through comparative tests that spiritual energy exists, Jonas and Crawford wrote, measurements for a healing presence ought to be "real-time, objective indicators rather than statistics," but their suggestion about putting random event generator (REG) devices in a laboratory or in intensive care unit to test for a healing presence, or detecting the intracellular calcium modulation across cell membranes "that would be expected to change when healing takes place," would leave ethicists aghast.[61]

According to Achterberg's hypothesis, prayer was to be considered as neither more nor less than mental telepathy, as an intervention. The literature review for the study included the early work done by Benson and others on transcendental meditation thirty years earlier. Also included in the early Benson studies were Tibetan monks meditating, Franciscan nuns praying, yoga practitioners, and twins, all relevant and important studies in research in mind-body medicine, and all of interest to neurologists.[62]

The flaws in Achterberg's study design raise a more universal problem of studying a healing presence or introspective rituals, which is always complicated by the presence of researchers. Hawaiian healers had been practicing their traditions for twenty-three years until Achterberg placed them in the "electromagnetically shielded control room and physically and optically isolated [them] from the receiver and scanner." Using magnetic resonance imaging, the study found "significant" activation of the brain that had to do with decision making, executive control (cingulated cortex), and the areas related to information processing (frontal lobes), as well as an area of the brain called the "precuneus," "about which very little is known." The authors concluded their study by questioning their findings. The presence of three researchers might have undermined the mechanism of the presence they were trying to measure; future research would need to examine the importance of empathy, and whether these findings "support previous research on distant healing suggesting that human intentions may directly affect others in ways that are not entirely understood."[63]

SCIENTIFIC PROTOCOLS

The research debate is about "effectiveness" of medical approaches and the best protocols in constructing and designing prayer research. Of course, all these studies can be criticized as flawed from the medical and the religious perspectives, because the presence of researchers may skew attempts to measure a healing presence. People who know they are "acting out" a religious practice will attain different levels of mental concentration than if they were not being observed. Given that artificially constructed prayer sessions may invalidate research results to the point that detractors call them "inconclusive," the finest minds in medicine are trying to build protocols that study how to measure "religiousness."

Much of the research measuring prayer begins with an acknowledgment that healers since ancient times used prayer as well as medicine. All boast merely "inconclusive" results. Jonas graded 130 studies in religion and spirituality as "good," all claiming 100 percent positive results though he gave them a D in "evidence level." Jonas ranked others even lower, from fair to poor, with a range of B, C, and F in evidence levels.[64]

Though few psychologists or psychiatrists "were interested in immunology" in 1969, Koenig and his associates at Stanford began to study the interaction of psyche and the immune system. As the field of psychoneuroimmunology developed during the 1970s, researchers looked at the ways in which the body's chemicals suppressed the immune system. The field gained further credibility in the 1980s as researchers proved that the endocrine system was "hard wired" to the central nervous system. Currently, according to Solomon, the "flood of information about the effects of immune cells on the brain (cytokins, neurohormones, neurotransmitters, neuropeptides) was precipitated by finding that these cells could signal the endocrine system and cause the body to "modify" its response to infections, tumors, and other diseased states. Solomon observed that all researchers in the 1970s and 1980s traced illness to stressors or life events such as birth, death, marriage, job loss, and Alzheimer's, concluding that long-term, unabated existence in the stress zone can cause illness.[65]

The variety, scope, and philosophy of research instruments for measuring religiosity remain highly controversial. Koenig and his respected associates used a standard protocol developed by Peter Hill and Ralph Hood, an instrument with 125 categories for defining religiosity.[66] Ten major factors have been used to categorize religiousness by Koenig and his associates, including denomination: researchers placed subjects into fifty-four categories for Christians, six for Jews, five for Muslims, three for Buddhists, two for Confucians, four for Hindus. The other categories included religious belief about whether there is a personal God and what image subjects have of God: a correlation has been demonstrated between high or low self-esteem and belief in God, as well as the variable of whether the Divine is perceived as stern and unforgiving or kindly and loving.[67] Additional factors in this instrument used to measure religiosity include: religious attitudes about one's faith as positive or negative. The degree to which the religious organization involves the individual in a social network or public religious activity is generally ranked as a positive factor by many cardiologists.

Other factors include multiple categories of private prayer time spent alone in religious activity. Koenig and Keith Maedor had a "six-frequency option," while others developed a "devotionalism scale" measuring prayer, habits of decision making, reading sacred or religious literature, and media use. Asking people point blank to rate the importance of religion was used to measure "religious salience." They also tried to measure first cause, or exactly why the subject was religious. In this effort, they tried to separate intrinsic motivation or philosophical principles from extrinsic motivators, separating the idea of religious orientation from self-interest.[68]

Intention, then, is as great a part of prayer as authenticity, whether distant or local, and "effectiveness" must be linked to depth of belief. But the difficulty of measuring authenticity of belief remains elusive despite the impressive refinements of the research instruments by Koenig and his associates. The "comfort factor" of leaning on God in times of distress seems easier to measure than asking if subjects had felt "they had ever been in the presence of God," another category of religiosity on the research instrument. Other affective experiences of God were offered as alternatives including fears of being punished by God, being afraid of God, and the like, and these also were factored into measurement. Most of these scales were developed during the 1960s and 1970s, but the utility of such categorization of "religiousness" that informed the first wave of researchers is being upheld by new, more exacting attempts to measure religious belief and habits of target populations today.

As scientific judgment matured about these measurements, life course and denominational choices were taken into account. For Jews, there was a six-to-ten item scale rating the maturity of beliefs about death and their knowledge of the Torah. For Hindus, a thirty-six-point scale assessed beliefs in traditions and practices. No scale has been developed specifically for Muslims, but the measures applicable to other faiths have been used, including measures of fear of death, and intrinsic versus extrinsic measures. For Buddhists, similar measures were employed, including those that rated anxiety.

Rabin and Koenig conclude that all the scales have some deficiencies. Today, researchers seem to think that each dimension of religiosity should be studied as a separate predictor, rather than trying to combine factors, so that greater specificity about religiousness would be more persuasive, leading to fewer sweeping generalizations about the impact of religion on health but to greater conclusiveness through a better research design.

Because the words "spirituality" and "religion" are nearly synonymous in the secular media marketplace, and mass media is far more comfortable with the term "spirituality" than with "religion," clinical researchers narrowed their use of the term "religion" so that it would be more specific. "The term spirituality is distinctive only if it involves a relationship with or search for the transcendent—however one defines the transcendent." Respected medical research among those involved in designing clinical trials, and in the education of doctors as well as in the practice of medicine, is attempting to demonstrate what doctors know intuitively and what they have observed from clinical experience. Measurements of well-being and cultural values, for example, on a nineteen-point scale that ranks items like the importance of faith, purpose in life, "mysticism subscales," and "participation in healing group," have been attempted but have not been used widely.[69]

Benson's INSPIRIT scale has been widely used since 1975: called "the Index of Core Spiritual Experience," his was far in advance of the work by Byrd or Harris. The INSPIRIT scale developed from a clinical trial of eighty-three medically ill adults over a ten-week period. INSPIRIT measured seven self-rated items that include in the definition of religiousness, "frequency of practices," a "feeling of closeness to a powerful spiritual force," having an "experience that God exists," and believing "that God dwells within the person."[70] Benson's INSPIRIT scale resembles Koenig's measurement of the intrinsic religiosity scale, which he argued was based on a 1967 scale developed by psychological researchers Allport and Ross.[71]

Koenig criticized another model called the FACIT (Functional Assessment of Chronic Illness) Spiritual Well-Being Scale, developed in Chicago during the 1990s. FACIT is constructed in two parts, measuring both Faith and Assurance and Meaning and Purpose. Koenig thought the instrument "contaminated" the scientific research reliability by correlating religion with mental health measurements.[72]

Happiness and religiousness are not, for scientific purposes, similar enough that the same tools can be used to measure both. Among those facing life-threatening illnesses, for example, Sloan-Kettering in New York developed a fifteen-point scale Systems of Belief Inventory. Not unlike Benson's INSPIRIT scale, Koenig concluded, categories that measure beliefs and practices are useful to the extent they also measure the "support received from one's religious community," which is particularly relevant for patients with serious medical illness. This is consistent with the widely accepted findings by many researchers in the fields of public health, gerontology, and social medicine that social support contributes to mental well-being and to physical health. The Fetzer Institute includes variables such as philanthropy, church volunteerism, the ability to forgive and forget, and silence.[73]

Given the number of times doctors have responded to studies published in the medical literature as being "inconclusive" based on "poor research design," Koenig's analysis is valuable. If the items "contaminated by this mental health" approach to religion were removed, the instrument would be more accurate: "Several of these other measurement scales would be fine, though they could still be vastly improved."[74] The difficulty of separating psychology from any study of mind-body medicine within the context of religion, and the inherent difficulty of measuring by any criteria what "religiousness" means, particularly in pluralistic cultures, will continue to challenge researchers.

AUTHENTICITY AND INTENTIONALITY

Research in medicine and religion is ultimately about the theological problem of suffering, its role in human spiritual growth, and how science might ameliorate suffering through scientific knowledge about health. Griffiths concluded that despite the many studies about how Eastern meditation reduces stress, generalizations by Western researchers are "difficult," for the obvious reason that clinical trials that ask religious people to perform practices "on demand" are not the same as more authentic rituals, which may influence outcomes.[75]

As Griffiths wrote in Koenig's edited volume of essays by leading researchers in the field, the Buddhist Four Noble Truths imply that while it is a high ideal to end suffering, the path to self-transformation is through suffering. Many religious traditions interpret suffering as positive, in the sense that it contributes to the ability to have compassion for others, and to a growth in wisdom. Nonetheless, "[w]e all want to be happy and to avoid suffering," as the Dalai Lama summarized.[76] Brown pointed out that the distinction between Eastern and Western traditions is not only their respective ideas about God, but also about the self in personal or impersonal relationship with God.[77] The "narrative" a patient "constructs" about his or her own spiritual history is "largely" the area "that physicians incorporate into the health care encounter."[78] As Brown observed, scientific reasoning "does not presuppose the exclusion of theology."[79]

The supernatural cannot very well be studied according to scientific investigation, and can only go so far as natural healing is discovered to be linked with the psychology of religious behavior. Many believers find ways to reconcile biology and beliefs: "The implications of psychoneuroimmunology and the faith factor are ambiguous enough to warrant caution on the part of both the medical and faith communities."[80] Finally, as Griffith, Brown, Koenig, Kaye, and many others conclude, for the practice of religion to yield a health benefit, the practitioner must actually believe, not just prescribe faith for the patient.

All this data is "correlational," rather than "causal," Koenig observed. Research about the correlation between religion and the immune system is not only recent; Koenig calls it "fledgling." Since the benchmark studies in the field by Byrd and by Harris were faulted for being

Christocentric, the term "prayer" is now used in its pluralistic context, as a practice communicating "with an absolute, immanent or transcendent spiritual force, however named. Such communication may take a variety of forms and may be theistic or nontheistic in nature, as in some forms of Buddhism."[81]

When scientists run clinical trials on heart patients in hospitals to test for the efficacy of prayer, consumers who have to make choices about their own health are interested in the results. Whether or not they pray or are religious, patients are looking for hope. That the negative results in the study by Benson ended up on the front page of the *New York Times* and in the monologue of late-night comedians the day before it was released by a medical journal raises a broader question about media in secular culture. Did the press pick up on this study because its results were negative?

The scientific data about health is hidden from the common reader because of the way in which journalists report on complex subjects. The press tends to "bookend" the debate about science and religion, reporting on conflict. With creationism, abortion, Terry Schiavo, and assisted suicide, the media emphasis is on birth and death. The objective surface of American news culture is political, and so those controversial moral issues are personified, profiling single individuals, feeding the collective consciousness with the idea that America is divided in its approach to health care—according to the red and blue states, between churchgoers and the unchurched—as if health were a partisan issue.

This division is constructed by media within the information economy, a "three-legged stool" that is comparable to that paradigm of the same name used by Benson to describe the way medicine should be practiced. In the case of the media, one leg of the proverbial stool is the pharmaceutical industry's role in advertising. The news media portrayal of an inherent conflict between science and religion obscures the far more compelling reality beneath, and that has to do with classes of people already battling diseases who are seeking healing through prayer, and the abundance of research data that correlates religious habits and health.

As advances in pharmacology continue to save lives, and the profits of Big Pharma soar globally, the evidence suggests that Americans want more than a pill from doctors—they want a healing presence, someone who will talk to them as a person who is more than a biological system. Bishop observed that when people are diagnosed with a terminal illness, when they ask "why," they do not expect a medical response.[82] Perhaps the traditional practice of medicine based on prescription drugs eventually will change because increasing numbers of Americans want to be treated "holistically," that is, as a biological system with a spiritual "mechanism" that is hard wired, inseparable from their overall state of health.

The leading edge of contemporary scientific inquiry is no longer defining how the mind affects the body when it perceives a threat, for that has been demonstrated time and again by Benson's generation, and is used as the base point for much subsequent research about religion and medicine by Rabin, McEwen, Sternberg, and many other distinguished neurologists, as discussed in the following chapter.

Much of the current research in the scientific literature has stayed safely on the side of the science of mind rather than venture into the science of the spirit, walking the fine line between behavioral psychology and the neurology involved in the stress response.

The role of prayer in healing remains as mysterious as ever, though more scientists today agree that healing can indeed be achieved through belief. This has led to a fascination with the impact of personality on the physical body rather than integrative theology. The clinical trials discussed here are about curing already diseased people postoperatively through prayer, not about calming the mind in order to prevent disease or maintain health. The latter is the prescription for meditation as part of mind-body medicine, the subject of the next chapter.

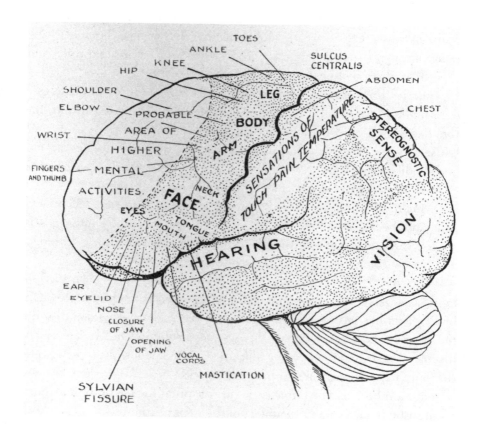

Figure 4.1: Special Brain Centers, *by William S. Sadler. From his book,* The Physiology of Faith and Fear *(Chicago: A. C. McClurg, 1912). Courtesy of the Newberry Library, Wing Collection Foundation.*

Chapter 4

BELIEF AND WELLNESS
MEDICAL PLURALISM AND HEALING

The systematic cultivation of healthy-mindedness as
a religious attitude . . . is anything but absurd.

—William James

The scientist who advocates religious explanations for healing is in a more tenuous position than the religious person who advocates science. The Dalai Lama used the word "secular" to describe the universal ethic needed in the new millennium, at a time when many people do not attend religious services and when membership in traditional religions is in decline. His Holiness used the word in one of his 240 books currently listed on Amazon.com, as one that would navigate between two key audiences endemic to the twenty-first century—those whose beliefs are embedded in a cultural niche that is religious in a sectarian sense, and those who do not believe in any religion, who see religion as part of the history of war and civil strife. We need a comparable, elastic vocabulary that hovers above sectarian belief, and that serves both those who talk about the role of religion in medicine and those in religion who put faith in science as an avenue to knowing about God as a healing presence. What we need is a comparable, "secular" bridging vocabulary that connects the contested space over religion and science that the mass media has created. Scientists at the Dalai Lama's Mind and Life Institute and at Harvard Medical School's Mind Body Institute (now at Massachusetts General Hospital) have made strides in the direction of creating such a vocabulary that bridges science and faith, and the same trend is going on in other places as well, including Duke University and Case Western Reserve's school of medicine. Meanwhile, the mass media has packaged the contemporary conversation about belief and wellness in multimedia products, best-selling books, instructional tapes, DVDs, and continuing medical education seminars, but this has only served to widen the opposition between how religions view science and how science views religion.

At the same time that an abundance of medical advice books have reached global audiences from best-seller lists, they have succeeded precisely because people who do not rely on religious authority tend to overestimate the value of medical authority. Distinguished medical educators have observed that physicians are "first of all healers."[1] But many religious people see themselves in the same way, namely Buddhist monks who meditate, Christian contemplatives, evangelical prayer groups engaged in intercessory prayer, and Christian Science prayer practitioners such as the followers of Rev. Eddy, who accepted her precept that "there were two avenues to an understanding of health—science and suffering."[2] As scientists research the connection between the emotions generated in the psyche, the biochemicals generated in the stress and relaxation responses in the mind, and physical healing, they have prescribed "mindfulness," incorporating meditation therapeutically in stress management techniques. In a separate body of literature demonstrating an understanding of the interconnections among mental, spiritual, and physical well-being, Tibetan and Trappist monks prescribed "awareness" and "listening," applying the language of a scientific diagnosis to the health of the soul.[3]

In classical mystical literature, the attitude toward suffering, or what St. John of the Cross called the "dark night of the soul," is that it is "essential to spiritual growth," and contemporary Buddhist and Trappist writers affirm a utilitarian attitude toward suffering.[4] Like his Buddhist friends, Trappist monk Thomas Merton saw a danger in the high ideas about prayer or contemplation that men imagine will help them "escape from a self."[5] Both Eastern and Western contemplative and meditative traditions argue that the way out of the self is inward: meditation and contemplation were roads to reach that reality.[6] "To pray is to know how to stand still and to dwell upon a word," according to the Rabbi Abraham Joshua Heschel.[7] The threshold of stillness is what doctors are using in mind-body medicine therapeutics to achieve the relaxation response and to get out of the anxiety of mind that causes the stress response. Stillness is not the same thing as mysticism, the deeper levels of knowing sought by those who give their lives over to the practices of meditation and contemplation in search of inner peace, happiness, and knowledge of the Divine Mind. This clarification needs to be made between those seeking inner transformation and those seeking wellness: one is universalist, the other utilitarian in their respective approaches to religion.

Given the difficulty of measuring the effectiveness of prayer in healing, how do the scientific and the religious views of suffering differ? From the religious standpoint, the crux of the problem is not how to avoid suffering, but how to understand what suffering has to teach about healing. From the medical standpoint, the investigation into prayer and meditation as therapeutic interventions constitutes a different way of thinking about healing in medicine with implications for how doctors see themselves. Among those in complementary and alternative medicine, prayer ranks among the top-ten most frequently used therapies, as reported by the CDC: 43 percent of Americans prayed for their own health, while 24 percent valued receiving prayers from others for their health.[8]

In the Western medical tradition, Drs. Harold Koenig, Herbert Benson, Larry Dossey, Bernie Siegel, and many others have multiple titles on the best-seller lists about how to live in wellness. The religious side of the contemporary investigation about the role of the mind in healing is as robust as that in the scientific literature. In some three hundred books currently in print by meditation and contemplative practitioners, the problem of suffering as a pathway to healing is analyzed from Eastern and Western, ancient and modern perspectives.

Much of this book is about how the finest scientific minds of our day have made recent discoveries about the impact of emotion and thought on the brain, which results in suffering. In complementary and alternative medicine, both prayer and meditation are used as therapeutic interventions to suffering. Though science and religion represent different avenues of knowing, as Bishop observed, the emerging body of knowledge about healing investigates how religion informs contemporary scientific debates.[9] As this chapter discusses, the genre of religious and medical advice books is a burgeoning media industry at the same time the formula for patient-provider communication lags behind what American consumers want, especially in terms of recognizing their spirituality as part of a holistic approach to biological medicine.

THE FAITH FACTOR

Religion has been used as a therapeutic intervention in Eastern medicine for centuries, in Buddhist, Chinese, and Indian cultures; but in American culture, attitudes toward religion in medicine have been treated separately, sometimes antagonistically. In India, Ayurveda that seeks health by "restoring the harmony" in the individual "is practiced at a national level within the federal health system," and traditional Chinese medicine is "often practiced in the same hospitals as conventional medicine."[10] In Japan the herb-based system of Kampo "is covered by the national health insurance plan and is practiced by many medical doctors."[11]

How religious factors such as prayer, belief, or other practices can work to buffer or reduce the physiological impact of the stress response is unknown. Rabin speculates that beliefs and the behaviors associated with religious and spiritual pursuits, beyond lifestyle measures, may contribute to "buffering the alteration of immune function by stress."[12]

Very few physicians other than Drs. Harold Benson and Jeff Dusek have studied Christian Scientists, a healthy cohort of religious individualists whose practices include daily reading and private prayer. Perhaps the historical image of the religion as an opponent of traditional medicine and prescription drugs discourages scientific study of how their beliefs correlate with their health. Daily reading of Eddy's *Science and Health*, not exactly an easy read, and their biblically based faith may put them on the margins of scientific study, because there are too many variables in the population, as the scant research that does exist suggests.[13]

Maybe the ethical problems of informed consent preclude the study of those who are ill and who claim healing through the ministrations of a healing presence of a practitioner who prays with the sick.

Over a four-month period in the winter of 1996–1997, Gallup polled Christian Scientists by telephone, a random sample, complicated by the religion constituting only 1 percent of the national denominational population. Further, available demographics about those who are in the religion are lacking. The target sample was to have two times as many nonmembers as members. The same questions were asked of all participants, about life satisfaction, health, the impact of their perceived health on their daily life, whether they smoked or drank, and their spiritual beliefs, and if they used traditional medicine or other treatments, physician visits, medications, or prescriptions. The results of the Gallup poll in the Benson-Dusek study showed that Christian Scientists were more satisfied with their life than the control group. More than one half of Christian Scientists (52 percent) confirmed they were very satisfied with their life, compared with only 37 percent of those who were not Christian Scientists; 71 percent of those in the church reported excellent or very good health, compared with 61 percent of the control group of non–Christian Scientists, made up of Protestants (39 percent), Roman Catholics (33 percent), and about 1 percent Jews, Muslims, Mormons, and Seventh-Day Adventists (1.8 percent). In the control group sampled by Gallup, there was only a 4 percent difference in their beliefs about the connection between religion and health: Christian Scientists reported 94 percent, all others 90 percent.

More than 80 percent of those surveyed by Gallup, in both groups, believed in the power of prayer, though attendance at religious services varied widely, from 62 percent of Christian Scientists to 46 percent of the control groups. While only 42 percent of the control group reported using mind-body medicine in the past year, two-thirds or 67 percent of Christian Scientists had done so, including megavitamins and homeopathy. The greatest difference, though, was about the use of personal prayer and meditation: 82 percent of Christian Scientists compared with 71 percent of all other religious groups reported that they prayed or meditated alone at least once a month. Both groups reported an equal number of visits to physicians if serious illness was involved.[14] Christian

Scientists were self-reported as being less, rather than more likely to exercise, watch cholesterol levels, and avoid sugar than the control group. Though this conflicts with the theories about religious attendance being equated with greater practice of self-care habits, it also raises a more important issue.

Scientific research has demonstrated that there is a "buffering" effect from religion among people already in a healthy state, a type of protection against the ravages of stress when that is inescapable. Yet the utility of belief as a buffer is an area difficult for science to investigate because it implies what Maedor objected to—a utilitarian approach to religious practices, to which believers ought to object.[15] Along with the issue of informed consent, the possibility of proving "conclusively" the "buffering" effects of religion raises ethical and theological problems. Given Madison Avenue's ability to sell a mix of religion and medicine in America's therapeutic culture, what might happen if an individual takes up the practices of a religious group precisely because they expect health outcomes promised by scientific research?

Clinical trials study not only the impact of prayer on the reduction of stress, but the effect of altruism and optimism on psychological well-being.[16] Rabin reported that out of one hundred studies in the literature, 79 percent reported a "significant positive association between religious involvement and well-being."[17] Lower mortality rates and better general physical and mental health were associated with people who belonged to a religion. As Solomon described in his study about religion and medicine, the separation between the two fields was a modern construction: the Bible is full of references to recovery from illness, only later did Western philosophy divide the mind from the body, and belief from wellness. Research about personality as a factor in the development of disease has focused not only the mind's role in the interpretation of events; the habits of thinking such as fears or anxiety; or supercritical voices, narcissism, or negative emotional states of any kind, but also on the mind's role in particular categories of diseases where the body turns on itself, such as autoimmune diseases.[18]

Researchers have tried to understand scientifically why religion is a factor in healing, and whether the mind becomes stressed because of disease, or whether the stress in the mind creates the disease. Though

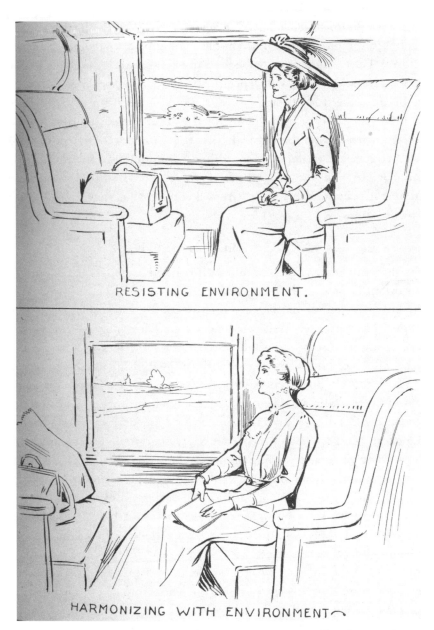

Figure 4.2: The Right and Wrong Way to Ride the Train, by William S. Sadler. From his book, The Physiology of Faith and Fear (Chicago: A. C. McClurg, 1912). Courtesy of the Newberry Library, Wing Collection Foundation.

hundreds of clinical trials have been conducted, the results are suggestive, but without definitive data that link religion and healing. Solomon
declared that the approach embedded in this research that tries to correlate personality type with specific types of diseases was inconclusive because the study designs were "flawed," and thus met with rightly
deserved "skepticism" from the medical establishment, a criticism that
reoccurs throughout the clinical literature about religion and medicine.[19] If religion buffers the mind-body interaction, maintaining the
mental peace that can keep the body in a steady state, the question
remains: if religion can reduce stress, keeping a person healthy, can it
help cure disease?

STRESS AND RELAXATION

Though many other respected and well-trained scientists have followed
the work of Benson and Koenig with additional research, these two men
were the founders of the late twentieth-century interest in their field,
though Sternberg and McEwen report that Hans Selye's work in the
mid-twentieth century first established the existence of the "stress effect"
on the mind and body.[20] Since the work in the mid-twentieth century by
Dr. Hans Selye, who introduced the fundamental term "stress response"
to mind-body medicine, scientific researchers have both proven and disputed at various times the relationship between mental stress and disease.
Like many people ahead of their time, Selye had to endure skeptics and
critics. In Selye's era, according to Sternberg, whose father was a medical
professor and physician and who knew Selye, "[t]he standard procedure
for identifying a new hormone involved making an extract—a kind of
soup or infusion—from any organ, often culled from the slaughterhouse."
Though initially Selye's findings were challenged by the medical establishment, Sternberg observed that "Selye's observations of the kinds of
white blood cells that increased and decreased in the course of stress
were accurate." More recently, under the leadership of Dr. Sternberg in
neuroimmunology at NIH, the stress response has been demonstrated in
random clinical trials with large data samples, down to the exchange of
oxygen at the cell level. In the late twentieth century, endocrinologists,
cardiologists, and neurologists especially have led the way in impressive
and conclusive research about the impact of emotions on health. Yet parts

of the deep brain still are mysterious even though neurologists know so much about where emotions come from in the brain.

Scientists are accomplishing interesting and impressive research proving that anxiety, stress, and negative emotions—anger, fear, depression, and grief—all have an impact on the messages that the mind sends to the body when the mind perceives a threat or worry. Sternberg's beautifully written book *The Balance Within*, a landmark work in medical literature, explains how the brain is a specialist emotionally, with different areas—an "ensemble of centers"—controlling positive and negative emotions. The part of the brain called the nucleus accumbens controls love, feelings of comfort, joy, and sexual responsiveness or "romantic" love. The part called the amygdala, two identical small almond-shaped parts on either side of the brain, controls fear, and its nerve fibers connect to the lower part of the brain, the hypothalamus, and brainstem, which "control breathing, sweating, heart rate, blood vessel and muscle tone." These lower parts of the brain also control sight, smell, hearing, taste, and other senses. Sternberg wrote, "The emotional centers, then, are wired above to incoming signals from the environment and below to motor centers, making us capable of responding to such signals at a moment's notice." All this happens "with split-second timing," she observed, "so emotions, in a very real sense, make us move." Even a scientist as learned and distinguished as Sternberg acknowledges that the brain still is mysterious, especially those parts that control memory.[21] Benson has made "remembered wellness" synonymous with "the placebo effect"; the status of remembered emotion is an aspect of the life of the brain that is still under investigation, especially by cardiologists and neuroimmunologists.

Each negative emotional state can lead to overproduction or underproduction of biochemicals that disrupt homeostasis, the body's harmonious state. McEwen describes, citing Sterling and Eyer, how "hormones act via receptors and set into motion changes at the cellular level, referred to as 'allostasis' . . . re-establishing stability through change." McEwen wrote that through "allostasis . . . the body re-establishes homeostasis in the face of challenge."[22] So the body accommodates the imbalanced state caused by emotions, and in so doing may create the conditions under which infections can occur because of a reduced immunity, and other diseased states that might result from the imbalance.

When the mind perceives an event as a stressor, the body's whole chemistry replies. When the mind perceives a threat it signals the body, provoking cells to interact in unnatural ways, that causes ill health. The depth of the emotional event causing major life changes—whether a death, a reversal of financial status, or a traumatic event such as a terrorist attack, tsunami, or hurricane—is a significant variable based on criteria of emotional impact. The second factor is how long the stress lasts: the "duration" of the trauma exacerbates the body's response. The central nervous system, the body's link with the brain, sends a signal not only to the organs of the body, but to the muscles, the skeleton, and the blood. All this physiological knowledge can be found in the scientific and popular literature of mind-body medicine, which is ranked by the National Institutes of Health as among the "alternative" approaches to medicine, though it is written about and studied by "regular" medical doctors as an established body of knowledge used in "complementary" or integrative practices, including neuroimmunology.[23]

As McEwen explained, the brain's stress response is immediate: the heart rate speeds; the homeostatic balance is disrupted; allostatic load causes the cells that were working in pairs to go haywire, repulsing rather than receiving; and the cells assigned to clean up bacteria are looking for a place to go. Even within the immune system, certain categories of cells act together, in pairs, to regulate each other's functions. If one half of the pair is affected by the pumping out of an imbalanced supply of hormone, it will throw off its paired receptor cell. Research has demonstrated that subjects under stress are less able to produce antibodies to fight a vaccination, and are more likely to contract an upper respiratory viral infection.[24] As mind-body medicine has popularized, and many advice books have traded on as common knowledge, neurochemicals appear in the blood "rapidly:" "catecholamines, epinephrine, norepinephrine." Each of these neurochemicals projects to different parts of the brain. Each affected part of the brain sends different signals to different organs of the body. The whole physical system is on alert, ready to fire, as soon as the brain perceives a threat.

Verrier and Mittleman correlated negative emotions and heart attacks, summarizing the studies of large populations: for example, 14 percent of fatal and nonfatal heart attacks among 270,000 people were preceded by emotional stress. Not only negative events caused this emotional stress leading to heart attacks, but also dreaming or replaying mentally the events that once provoked emotional distress could cause myocardial infarction.

Anger is far more likely to lead to death from heart failure than physical exertion: the effect of exertion lasts less than one hour, but anger's effects last two hours. Verrier cites Kubzansky's studies in 1997 on how worry, a dimension of anxiety, contributes to aging. The connection between mental states and the sympathetic nervous system, which affects the heart, also has an impact on blood platelets, affecting the clotting factor.[25]

Until recently, mental stress—especially from financial strain among the elderly, domestic disharmony, and particularly anger—were not understood as integral to a holistic approach to the body's tolerance for its psychosocial environment. Psychology and psychiatry long were separate from neurology, but contemporary medicine is not only pluralistic, it is interdisciplinary. Researchers have demonstrated that whether a body is healthy or becomes diseased depends on its ability to control the mind and its negative or positive thoughts: the interpretation of events and the mental processing of affective perceptions create the emotions that cause the mind to disrupt the heart, lungs, and all internal organs.[26]

Although common knowledge, Harvard's Mind Body Institute and leading NIH neurologists repeat how different hormones react in the same way that they did when the bodies of cavemen fought off intruders, the brain telling the body to fight or flee, to rest, or to run in self-preservation.[27] That once served a purpose in prehistoric times of course, but today the threat is imagined. In media speak, we talk about threats as constructed, imaginary, and political—much of it relayed by "hyper" media through the Internet, saturation television advertising, and twenty-four-hour news channels that emphasize crises. Human emotions today are overtaxed, continuing to work within the brain even when the body is not threatened physically but virtually through messages in mass media. Without awareness of the unreality of these threats, how can people control their emotional response? Even at that, the widespread violence reported by the news in urban areas, the violence in film, as well as psychological fears that visually absorbing such images can set off, could hypothetically provoke the same stress response. So one can see that the external communication environment as well as political factors such as violence in the news, in photojournalism, and in the telecommunication of bombing, suicides, executions, or terrorist beheadings run on the Internet—which fill our mass media because of the political realities of our day, however remote geographically—have an impact on our public health. Scientific research has yet to test if the emotional center of the brain makes the distinction between threats at a distance and threats in proximity. Do the emotional centers of the brain triggered in the stress response also differentiate among print, visual images, commercial messages, fiction, and actual, though geographically remote, events in the news?

The mind that perceives a threat triggers a mechanism in the brain so that neural pathways and hormonal centers release substances as neuroscience has established. Medical doctors have long known that stress occurs from within the psychology of the mind as well as from the uncontrollable externalities of life events in family and jobs, war and catastrophe. Stress triggers disease in a very complex but scientifically demonstrable way. The reverse of the stress response, the calming effects of prayer, has been investigated by medical science. The calm mind is different. Science has demonstrated with the aid of magnetic resonance imaging what parts of the brain are activated when contemplating different types of affective states, such as compassion and peace. The studies about the impact of mental peace, which is to say studies about wellness, are in their infancy as the scientists engaged in this research have described.

In order to demonstrate the power of the mind to calm or to create stress that affects the body, magnetic resonance imaging has been used to show graphically and in color how the mind changes when thoughts change. Thoughts about compassion, for example, "color" different parts of the brain. To demonstrate this visually, researchers have attached electrodes to the skulls of transcendentalist meditation practitioners, and they have done the same with Tibetan monks whose bodies can dry wet sheets with their warmth while meditating.

Beyond the exotic element in studies about contemplative monks, there are other, more ordinary approaches to explaining why a calm

mental state is important for the health of the body. Life course studies have been conducted among professed religious, nuns, monks, and
priests about submission to a higher power, which resulted in a lower
degree of stress. Buddhists such as Thich Nhat Hanh and the Dalai
Lama, have talked about the average American living as if in the midst
of an "anxiety pandemic."[28] The Mind Body Institute has incorporated
Eastern meditation styles of calming the mind, with common Western
approaches to behavioral medicine, addressing forgiveness, as well as
weight management, mother-child relationships, life-mapping, "mini"
meditation sessions of five minutes, yoga, and stress management as
part of on-going health education.

Undoubtedly, because of the life work of the eminent physicians Dr.
Harold Benson and Dr. Herbert Koenig, who also teach medicine, many
future doctors will be able to attend courses on spirituality and medicine as they attain their M.D. degrees. Dozens of centers for the study
of alternative medicine have been established within or in association
with leading medical academies. Drs. Koenig and Benson have both
published countless journal articles and numerous best-selling books
and have received considerable media attention. Benson's trademark *The
Relaxation Response* and Harvard's Mind Body Institute emphasize meditation. Jon Kabat-Zinn, a psychology professor, has adapted this at the
University of Massachusetts–Amherst for patients with heart disease.
His book, *Full Catastrophe Living*, picked up Benson's prescriptions for
calming the cardiovascular system through meditative style habits: both
he and Richard Davidson are founding board members of the Mind and
Life Institute, working with the Dalai Lama to integrate Buddhist principles about mental training and behavioral science research into the
impact of mental peace on physical health.[29]

POSITIVE AND NEGATIVE THOUGHT

Mathieu Ricard, Ph.D., abbot of Shechen Monastery, said in a recent
meeting of the Mind and Life Institute that meditation or "mental training" can be used to strengthen the mind "so that we are living our life
in the most optimal way."[30] From the Buddhist viewpoint, Ricard said
that "mental health is not just the absence of mental illness." From his
perspective, the way that many Americans go about their life is best

described as a "widespread pandemic," full of emotional highs and lows, and moving at such a pace that the "mental state is noticed less and less." Attentiveness to the mental state is the key to the mental training that is the purpose of meditation, and awareness within the meditative state allows one to assess whether the mind is wandering, spinning, and full of distracting thoughts or negative emotions.[31]

Buddhists believe that "we all want to be happy and free from suffering."[32] Freedom from suffering opens up the mind to the possibility of compassion. Though it has only recently been integrated in the medical knowledge, compassion is valued by Buddhists, Christians, and many other religious traditions. In his summary of Buddhism's principles, Ricard said that in order for the mind to be in a state of compassion, the "mental toxins of hatred, nagging desire, jealousy" must be cleansed through the practice of meditation or mental training. In other words, negative emotions keep the mind in a state of distortion, dominated by habit, and in a state of dis-ease that is not optimal mental health. "Mental health is not just the absence of mental illness," according to Ricard. "Our whole goal is to free ourselves and others from suffering. Compassion can emerge from understanding the interdependence with others and cultivating emotional balance. . . . There cannot be outer peace without inner peace."[33]

At the same meeting, Ajahn Amaro, coabbot of Abhayagiri Buddhist Monastery, outlined the main principles and reasons for mental training. Offering his ideas "not as dogma" but merely as ideas to consider; he described *dukkha*, the suffering that comes from dissatisfaction, as the type of suffering that the mind creates. This is distinct from physical pain or catastrophic events. The quality of the mind that is of concern to Buddhists is its ability to "lose its balance" or get "caught up in worry," even about things that will never happen or don't exist, as Amaro described at length. "The Four Noble Truths are cast in classical Indian medical diagnosis," he said. "Physicians exist because we don't experience health all the time," explained Amaro, "nor do we experience happiness all the time."

The Buddhist idea of suffering, *dukkha*, or dissatisfaction has two dimensions: first, the suffering that is part of being human; second, "adventitious suffering," the mental pain of anxiety that the mind adds to reality. Many people try to escape mental pain through the senses, causing further suffering to the body through addictions. Acceptance of suffering, whether grief, catastrophic loss, or physical pain, diminishes the *dukkha*, according to Amaro. Meditation takes the rhythms of the body, particularly the breath, as its metronome, to "refine the innate abilities we already possess . . . and by focusing the attention on the breath, break the habit of mind that constantly creates scenarios for the future or rewrites the past," according to the abbot. "Meditation is learning how to think and how not to think," he said, "not how not to be drawn into compulsive cycles." It has been said that all babies are born into a state of the bliss that Buddha describes was innate in us all, and that all of the rest of life is a forgetting of that bliss and a movement slowly toward death and then rebirth. But Buddhist bliss is not "being zoned out" but is a state of mental alertness, or awareness, an ability to "relate compassionately with all other beings that suffer because we ourselves know what it is to have suffered." Amaro's prescription for the definition of mental health is a mental peace, an "easefulness," an enlightened awareness about our motivations and habits, without compulsions. But within Western psychology, Amaro observed, Buddhism is considered "less than sane."[34]

Pema Chödrön's advice in *When Things Fall Apart*, for example, argues that the Buddhist principle of impermanence can help alleviate mental suffering by helping people to see how the fear of death is the motivation for their restless discomfort that leads to stress: "We're all addicted to hope—hope that doubt and mystery will go away. . . . When we feel suffering, it doesn't mean that something is wrong. . . . Suffering is part of life." Modern culture is a "babysitter," in Chödrön's view, for what many Buddhists refer to as the modern condition—that is, a "widespread anxiety and panic" about suffering that might happen in the future. Buddhists prescribe awareness of the present as an antidote to such anxiety. As the following chapter discusses, when it comes to mental health, a case can be made that the pandemic of anxiety is fed by the media, which often communicate fear in order to encourage listeners to "stay tuned."

From the perspective of a Buddhist woman monk like Chödrön, the relaxation from anxiety comes with the awareness that everything is changing all the time, that physical states of youth and health, too, are impermanent. But many "unenlightened" ones, she would argue, spend a lifetime resisting biological science and in fear of death. "Impermanence is a principle of harmony," she wrote. "When we don't struggle against it, we are in harmony with reality. Many cultures celebrate this connectedness. There are ceremonies marking all the transitions of life from birth to death, as well as meetings and partings. . . . Our suffering is based on our fear of impermanence." Chödrön summarized the Buddhist views that suffering needs to be countered within the reality that everything has its opposite, so pain and pleasure, birth and death, inspiration and aridity, are all part of life. If meditation or mental training leads to an understanding of how everything is always in transition, then the periods of suffering would be lessened and pain decreased, with the understanding that these are waves in a sea of time. If impermanence is understood, not feared, it is recognized as part of the cycle of life. "Nothing ever goes away until it has taught us what we need to know," in the view of Buddhist practitioners.[35]

The purpose of meditation for Buddhist practitioners is to gain greater insight and clarity about reality, about the self, and about thoughts as impermanent. As many popular books by Buddhist monks such as Nhat Hanh, Chödrön, Amaro, and others assert, being "gentle or friendly with the Self is a kindness" that results from what Buddhists call Big Mind, which can be compassionate because it sees and understands the frailty of all people, that we are all mortal and vulnerable in some degree, both emotionally and physically. As for managing negative or toxic emotion—the anger that science has demonstrated ravages the cardiovascular system in the stress response—the Buddhist view is to use meditation first to accept the anger, which is the result of inflicted pain we cannot control or in some cases reply to, and turn down the reaction by turning up the meditation about compassion, emptiness, and impermanence, all the concepts in Buddhism that contribute to the understanding that enemies can become friends. Meditation teaches how to observe the self, as if standing outside and looking at the self. The point and purpose of meditation, then, is not as a stress reducer or a therapeutic intervention so that people can continue to hope. As in contemplative traditions, among meditators, there are levels of the private practice that lead to different depths of insight. "Mini-meditation," the therapeutic intervention at the

Mind-Body and Stress Relaxation centers in Massachusetts, has helped to reduce anxiety and stress and is helpful for cardiac patients as well as others. In the Buddhist view, relaxation is not the point, awareness of reality is. Just as with prayer practices, the therapeutic use of mediation frames the practice as a medical commodity.

Thich Nhat Hanh wrote in his contemporary classic, *Being Peace*, that "Suffering is not enough. We must also be in touch with the wonders of life. They are within us and all around us, everywhere, any time," and "we are more than our sorrow." Employing the media as an analogy, the Vietnamese Buddhist compared human beings to a television set with millions of channels, who should not let one dominate. "If we turn the Buddha on, we are the Buddha. If we turn sorrow on, we are sorrow. . . . We have the seed of everything in us, and we have to . . . recover our sovereignty. . . . Practicing meditation in this kind of society is very difficult. We have a thousand things, tapes and music, to take us away from ourselves. . . . To meditate means to be aware of what is going on."[36]

In the Christian contemplative tradition, Christian monks describe a comparable layer of awareness achieved through depth and duration of practice, sometimes using the same language, sometimes using the language of grace. Writer and Trappist monk Thomas Merton, who was very close to his Buddhist counterparts before his untimely death in 1968, described the ecumenical "sapiential" experience—that is, a knowing about reality, the "deepest and most authentic fruit" of the interiority practice. Merton defined contemplation as "the direct intuition of reality . . . awareness . . . that presupposes the knowledge and practice of certain traditional disciplines." The ability to sit, to be still, and to contemplate are "gifts," according to Merton, and "routine exercises of piety and a few external acts of worship and service performed as a matter of duty" because the individual wants to "insure" himself or herself may be prescribed as therapeutic in a clinical sense, but the sacred and medical are two very different levels of the practice. As Merton observed, though contemplation may be used as a therapeutic, it is useless if the individuals' "minds and hearts are taken up with their own ambitions and troubles and comforts and pleasures and all their worldly interests and anxieties and fears."[37]

Kabat-Zinn, who serves on the board of the Mind and Life Institute, noted that "stress is not used as a synonym for dukkha" and that hospitals are "dukkha magnets," a good environment to investigate suffering. Stress reduction clinics, such as the one he founded at the University of Massachusetts–Amherst, address "the needs of people who have long-term stress that medical intervention has been unable to reduce."[38] Yet he acknowledged that mindfulness-based stress reduction is consistent with the central principles of Buddhist meditation, a "moment to moment nonjudgmental awareness cultivated purposefully by paying attention to the present moment." Yet meditation as Buddhist monks practice it, for whole days at a time, is a key to greater self-knowledge, not the medical approach to improving cardiovascular health.

In both Eastern and Western contemplative traditions, the longer the practice, the deeper the knowledge of self and awareness of reality: lowering blood pressure may be a side effect, but sitting for long hours is not physically comfortable nor initially an easy posture. The greatest act of compassion, Kabat-Zinn observed, echoing the Buddhist writers Chödrön, Hanh, and others from the contemplative tradition, is for each individual to observe what is going on in both the body and the mind and to live in the present: "do not rewrite the past or the future," they prescribe. Kabat-Zinn termed the meditation practices the "training wheels" for sixteen thousand patients who used his clinic between 1980 and 2005, with beneficial effects on their cardiovascular system and heart disease. The stress-reduction therapeutic intervention also uses poetry and guided imagery, the types of practices initiated by Benson and others such as Kabat-Zinn associated with behavioral medicine, stress reduction, psychoneuroimmunology, and endocrinology.

Richard Davidson, a professor of psychology at the brain research center at the University of Wisconsin–Madison, also a founding member of the Mind and Life Institute, pointed out that people have different levels of happiness, and those levels are related to emotional skills that can be learned through mental training. "Differences in happiness can be associated with different patterns of brain function," as his research demonstrated, and the emotions that are governed by neural circuitry exist in a two-way relationship with the body. "When we change the brain we change the body," he said. Neurogenesis, the process by which the brain can rebuild itself, is central to the thinking that informs Davidson's scientific research and to meditative stress-reduction practices, both of which show that exercise can promote rebuilding the brain and that stress can reduce its ability to rebuild itself. People who can control their negative emotions "show a steeper decline in cortisol," and meditation "strengthens the cortical regulatory circuitry that modulates the limbic system," Davidson said.[39]

Depression is the "common cold of mental disorders," and depression rates in the United States are about 10 percent of the population, second only to heart disease in terms of its costliness to society, according to Zindal Seagal, a professor at the University of Toronto. Scientists are interested in the impact of stress on the brain's ability to get along with itself, and in how meditation, which has been demonstrated to sharpen the brain's neural activity, can be used to lessen depression, which science has demonstrated is caused in part by stress.[40]

Depression is not *dukkha*, nor is it sadness or unhappiness, because scientists really do not understand depression fully, as neuroscientists have explained. Some people cannot control their depression, and they can slip back into depression even after eighteen months in remission. "The one thing we can control is our reactivity to sad thoughts," according to Seagal, and some people have "an emotional tenderness for the sad thoughts of the past, so they have a tendency to get back into that sadness, almost through an affection for the same memories." Cognitive therapy is more effective than medication, in Seagal's view. Mindfulness teaches a way of managing moods, "teaches patients recovery by intensifying their awareness," Seagal said.[41]

B. Alan Wallace, founder of the Santa Barbara Institute and a former Tibetan monk and graduate of Stanford in religious studies, describes Eudaimonic well-being as an ideal state, a "way of being where flourishing, inner happiness, truth and virtue are not contingent upon pleasant things happening to you." Developing generosity and compassion were part of the cultivation phase of this Eudaimonic state of wellness. "Genuine happiness is liberation," Wallace said, and the sense of wellness that springs from within can happen in times of adversity. "Even in illness, people can flourish, even in the face of death," Wallace said. "Dharma is the well-being that comes from living ethically, mental balance and the exploration of the consciousness that leads to spiritual flourishing or eudomonia."[42]

Ralph Snyderman, dean of medicine at Duke and coauthor of popular books with Andrew Weil, concluded that the "portions of the brain that control compassion can minimize the part of the brain that causes fear and anxiety." Through mental training, habits of negative emotions that create stress and that can lead to disease and mental illness or depression can be reversed but not cured. "Mindfulness based stress reduction can be applied to large numbers of people, not just monks or religious people, but the applications of meditation can treat an area of disease."[43] Scientists could reach these goals by understanding that science is only one source of knowledge—if the science community also practiced mental training, Snyderman concluded.[44]

THE HEALING INTENTION

A physician observed that medicine's failure to respond to patient needs for knowing about religious questions has driven patients to complementary and alternative practitioners, where patients may run the risk of getting information about medicine from those whose bias is toward religion.[45] This opinion is borne out by survey statistics offered by Schoenberger and others. In a recent survey mailed to 7,479 physicians, nurses, and physical and occupational therapists, the majority of the 1,200 (17 percent) who responded to the survey regarded prayer as a "legitimate health care practice," yet most health professionals would probably be more comfortable with the word "meditation" rather than "prayer." Of all the health professionals polled, physicians were the least likely to discuss prayer. More nurses or therapists than physicians used either prayer or meditation in their professional health practice. Though many physicians reported that they prayed and meditated daily, most did not "refer their patients for meditation or religious consultation."[46]

"Short of prescribing religion," Dr. Harold Koenig questioned his peers, what "can a physician do" in clinical practice to address the patient's need for religious concerns where they exist? Koenig stopped short of telling doctors to actually prescribe prayer, an act that he would consider intrusive, no matter what the scientific evidence. If a doctor is sensitive to the patients' concerns, she or he would regard the topic of religion as one where the physician could too easily overstep the medi cal role, treading on the chaplain's turf. He argued that the safest course would be to take a patient's spiritual history, something that less than 10 percent of doctors do, according to Koenig.[47]

After all, not everyone thinks about religion as a comfort. For some, religion is a source of anger or fear, anxiety, or dread, all feeding stress. The most recent research published in 2006 on this subject concludes that, among doctors, "only half bring up" the subject of religion.[48] The purpose of a physician taking a patient's spiritual history is to find out where the patient is on the spectrum of attitudes toward religion, and if the idea itself might create stress. Equipped with such a history, the physician could understand whether religion could help the patient cope, whether the church or other religious institution was a source of social support, and whether their image of God was a comfortable one. Many doctors do not talk with patients about spirituality because they are uncomfortable with the communication aspects of talking about issues that touch so profoundly on the question of spiritual identity—where each person is on their respective path. Koenig wrote that seriously ill patients have many spiritual needs that are unmet, and that doctors ought to discern whether the patient wants to speak with a chaplain, attend a religious service, or have someone to pray with. "Although physicians may not be able to personally address these spiritual needs, they can be sure someone else does." The downside of physician involvement in prescribing prayer, he argued, is that the focus shifts from the patient to the doctor, and "you run the risk of coercion." However, when terminal illness or serious surgeries are involved, doctors ought to learn their patients' perception and "sincerely try to understand their worldview." When religion conflicts with prescriptions, transfusions, or other interventions in conventional medical care, he urged, it becomes even more important to understand patients' spiritual histories.[49]

The problem of how doctors can better communicate with patients is an interdisciplinary communication field in itself, but Schmidt addressed the implications for the clinical professional in a way that bridges the CAM literature and the work of the leading neurologists, with relevance for those interested in better patient-provider communication.[50] If Schmidt's recommendations for healing health care environments were extended to the organization of hospitals and the national health care system, including the insurance and pharmaceutical industry, the rec-ommendations would be transformational. His prescription for medita-tion, if prescribed for prayer, would border on the type of "intrusive" or "aggressive" dialogue with patients that Koenig cautions against, based on decades of medical practice and knowledge of the research to date.

Schmidt strikes at the crux of the matter, though, by transferring to the doctors the Buddhist concepts of mindfulness embedded in the development of stress-reduction and mind-body therapeutics. The role of the doctor or health care professional is to "elicit self-healing powers" in the patient, he argued, echoing Benson and many others. Schmidt wrote that the healer's attitude toward the patient is the key to unleash-ing this power of religion or spirituality in medicine. If it has been dem-onstrated since ancient times in folk medicine, and a century ago in Rev. Eddy's claims that a healing presence can do more good than medicine, Schmidt's challenge suggests doctors need to become that healing pres-ence. He argued that "the healing intention" is vital to the process of patient-provider communication. The stickler is whether the doctor is the healing presence patients require.

In many cases in twenty-first-century medicine, it is not just the patients who need healing, whose dissatisfaction with conventional med-icine has created the consumer-driven mega-shift toward integrative practices. Doctors themselves need to be healed; Schmidt asserted that "healing the healers" would transform the practice of modern medicine. By this he means doctors need to practice what they preach. Even Benson admitted that only recently did he employ the meditative practices of mindfulness that he had been prescribing for patients for decades.

Mindfulness is the path through which mind connects to mind, and so the doctor could exude the compassion that the patient needs to feel: "Compassion connects the suffering of the patient with the healer's own suffering, and this emotional connection instantiates the healing rela-tionship."[51] Schmidt argued that the healing intention is crucial to the healing presence that helps the patient to realize he or she is being cared for, diminishing fears and anxieties and contributing to the "coping" physiological mechanism that Koenig described in clinical trials and observed on an individual basis. The core of the Healing Intention begins when the health care professional encounters wellness as well as illness. Self-acceptance and self-love on the part of the provider as well as patient play a vital role in the physiology of the healing process.[52]

The literature of contemplation and meditation draws the distinction between being and doing, important to the concepts of religious knowledge in both Eastern and Western traditions. The problem with prayer as a therapeutic intervention is that it can be perceived by doctors as something else to "do" rather than "being" with the patient in compassion. By arguing that the doctor should concentrate on being rather than doing, Schmidt is making the case for the "inner attitude of the professional" that can shape how the healer's questions communicate themselves to the patient, through tone as well as verbal and nonverbal behavior. When a patient has identified with his or her illness, the tone and style of communication from provider to patient can alter how a question is heard.[53] Schmidt observed that the doctor needs to communicate to the patient a spiritual attitude of unconditional love, acceptance, and positive regard, and this cannot occur when the healer has not yet developed that dimension of mindfulness. The role of humor and laughter has been documented in the mind-body literature as therapeutic, but when applied to the healing presence of doctors, the humor needs to be more subtle, and to communicate the mystic's message that "all will be well," even in the face of serious illness—that the doctor is not judging the patient in any way, but accepting the sufferer as someone who once was well, just like the doctor is today. Among older patients, many of whom are under stress, depressed, and self-conscious about the appearance of their bodies, for example, the doctor needs to treat them as if they were young and had many years ahead to live. An attitude of unconditional love is free from judging the illness or the patient in any negative way—a quality of health practitioners that the Buddhist literature explains, and which Schmidt summarizes succinctly. Acceptance of the patient's reality and the ability to separate the patient from the illness that he or she is carrying are attributes of a physician's healing presence.

Schmidt's depiction of how a doctor's stress or lack of mindfulness can communicate itself to the patient is realistic. He hypothesized in describing that "the doctor is mentally preoccupied with the patient's medical history and with choosing a possible diagnosis, while he or she is, at the same time, listening to the patient. His mind is not with the patient but elsewhere; the doctor is busy thinking in the past (medical history) or future (therapy to be described)."[54]

To transform that model, the mindful practitioner would give each patient his or her entire attention while they are together. The patient ought to leave the communication encounter in the clinic with the feeling that he or she is cared about, thought about positively no matter how old or how ill, that the doctor will remember the patient and accept him or her as is, and that the doctor is not too busy, tired, or stressed out by other patients to think about him or her as an individual, rather than part of a herd. "Mindfulness is a way of being," Schmidt observed.[55] Schmidt contends, and convincingly so, that it is not enough that the patient believes, prays, and meditates. The healer must also practice in faith.

Schmidt advocated a training program for practitioners modeled on the stress reduction protocols at Harvard and the University of Massachusetts. Such a course would lead health care providers in a series of reflections about their motivations for being in health care, their own beliefs, limits, social skills, and meditation practices. Schmidt took it one step further, arguing that an "Optimal Healing Environment" would apply compassion and mindfulness not only through the individuals encountering patients, but through small groups, integrating the latest findings from integrative medicine to reframe the daily habits of the place itself so that it is increasingly patient-centered and aware of their needs.[56]

Luskin doubted whether practices such as meditation that originated within spiritual contexts can be distilled from their ethnic roots and used as a medical intervention.[57] The threshold of the practice is calming the mind, breathing, and concentrating, all of which serve the body's cardiovascular system, but it takes years of meditative practice to achieve a level of "no self," or the ego-less state advocated by the Dalai Lama. Luskin is more impressed with the positive virtues than the practices extracted from faith traditions, as long-term solutions to the "transformation" that is at the heart of every religion, and of prayer or meditation, and for therapeutics in mind-body medicine.

Transformation heals more than the body; it changes the mind in order to unite the spirit-body-mind. Luskin reports that forgiveness and other virtues, including positive thinking, are skills that patients can learn, just as they learn new styles of meditation or prayer. More research will be required to demonstrate the link between "transformative" practices and skills such as gratitude, forgiveness, compassion, and hope, though they are being investigated through research in positive psychology for their connection to mind-body medicine.

MEDIA AND THE DALAI LAMA

Just as the physician today needs to be able to communicate with patients about their deeper beliefs, so do monks have to be able to communicate about science, often working with or through the media coming to a clearer sense of how the media devalues belief in favor of consumer materialism as a cult of reality. No one does this better today than the Dalai Lama, a healing presence for many seeking to bridge the inner world of spirituality and the empirical study of brain science.

As part of his ten-day tour of America in November 2005, the Dalai Lama delivered the keynote address to the twenty thousand assembled scientists at the annual meeting of the Society for neuroscience, following Mind and Life Institute discussions on November 8–10, 2005. The media attention focused on protests against his appearance, though his actual keynote address received little attention. The *Washington Post* reported on the "pushback" from the Dalai Lama's ten-day tour in America. Ever a popular celebrity, his appearances routinely draw thousands, so anything negative about the Dalai Lama would constitute "news." Petitions were circulated, according to the media report, protesting the appearance of a spiritual leader giving an hourlong keynote address to a scientific society. The *Washington Post* wrote that a group of Chinese American researchers circulated a petition, gathering six hundred signatures, asking that the appearance be cancelled. The group also wrote letters to the editor and editorials in *Nature*.[58] The *Post* noted that the six hundred signatures of protest were not only Chinese. "Inviting the Dalai Lama to lecture on 'neuroscience of meditation' is of poor scientific taste, because it will highlight a subject with largely unsubstantiated claims and compromise scientific rigor and objectivity at a prestigious meeting. . . . The presentation of a religious symbol with a controversial political agenda may cause unnecessary controversies, unwanted press, and significant divisions among SFN members from multiple geographic locations, and with conflicting religious beliefs and political leanings," according to the language of the petition.[59]

Counterprotesters gathered more signatures supporting his appearance. When the Dalai Lama did speak, it was anticlimactic from the media's standpoint. Yet the occasion of his delivering "Science at the Crossroads" was a historic occasion. In his hour-long address, the Dalai Lama made the case for the work of neuroscientists who were moving beyond the academic understanding of their field to connect with humanity and to address questions of "urgency" that will have "profound benefits" for humanity and "deepen our basic understanding of what it means to be human."[60] He compared the scientist with the "science of meditation." The Dalai Lama said that "both Buddhism and modern science share a deep suspicion of any notion of absolutes, whether conceptualized as a transcendent being, as an eternal, unchanging principle such as soul, or as a fundamental substratum of reality. Both Buddhism and science prefer to account for the evolution and emergence of the cosmos and life in terms of the complex interrelations of the natural laws of cause and effect. . . . Both traditions emphasize empiricism." Exploring the common ground between research science and a spiritual science, the Dalai Lama described the two levels of the science of meditation, the first stilling the mind, the second developing the understanding. He cautioned the scientists not to make sweeping assumptions about meditative practices, so that both "parties in the dialogue can find the common ground of empirical observable facts."[61]

Finally, the Dalai Lama raised the need for a "secular ethic." By that he did not mean to discount what is held to be religious or sacred but to connect the scientist and the science of meditation with his often-repeated theme on the search for happiness, an end to suffering, and everyone's responsibility to the larger society. Scientists need to do more than "further scientific knowledge and enhance technological power," leaving the political choices to the individual, he said. The "secular ethics" he endorsed is one that embraces "key ethical principles, such as compassion, tolerance, a sense of caring, consideration of others, and the responsible use of knowledge and power—principles that transcend the barriers between religious believers and non-believers."[62]

His argument for the relationship between science and Buddhism—and by extension between brain research, meditation, clinical medicine, and prayer—is based in the "interconnectedness" of all humanity. Whether it is the electronic media or the global economy, international tourism or the environment, he concluded, the world is increasingly interconnected. "Like the fingers of the hand, connected at the palm," to employ the Dalai Lama's metaphor, are science, ethics, religion and nonreligion, and Eastern and Western medicine interconnected.[63]

MEDICAL ADVICE AS A SPIRITUAL COMMODITY

While medical science has devoted itself to "proving" the positive impact of faith and belief in health in a body of scientific literature, and in a raft of best-selling self-help advice books by physicians, one can see the dangers of the commodification process caused by popularizing medical ideas that contain religious elements.

Modern medicine has taken Ralph Waldo Emerson's self-reliance to the edge in a body of knowledge about self-healing. It "matters very little" whether meditation or prayer "works" as a therapeutic intervention because the "instrumental" and "contractual" relationship implied by the utility of religion in therapeutic medicine thrusts Buddha or God into the marketplace of an economy of self-centered commodities, as Keith Maedor, a theologian-physician affiliated with Duke University's Divinity and Medical School, objected.[64]

Dr. Maedor responded to the late twentieth-century movement in faith-based religious intervention that interprets and applies the spiritual principles of Buddhism or Christianity in a therapeutic context, in which meditation or prayer is used for the benefit of an individual's health. Maedor wrote, "God is not so much the one who wills the health of God's creatures as a sign of God's care for the creation, as the one whose will is bound instrumentally by and to the logic of exchange. . . . God becomes obligated to fulfill the contract by providing health in exchange for devotion." Maedor calls the problem of "locating and describing God" part of the modernist and postmodernist dilemma.[65] Whether people think about God as local or "non-local," to borrow the phrase from the medical science literature, is the tip of the eschatological iceberg.

Maedor observed that

> God is defined by the logic of exchange as a producer of desirable
> commodities to be exchanged as a matter of course for particular
> kinds of devotional behaviors, such as prayer, meditation or church
> attendance. Now, understood within the contexts of several religious
> traditions from and within which they typically are engaged . . . such
> religious behaviors are properly understood as practices. . . . Within
> the logic of exchange . . . devotional behaviors are reduced, in effect,
> to techniques. Techniques are forms of action that are expected to
> produce specific, objective results that are external and instrumental
> to the actions themselves. . . . Practices . . . are internal to the ways of
> life in which they are embedded. . . . The primary point of practices is
> the activities themselves and the kind of person they form, while the
> primary point of techniques is the immediate results they produce for
> the person employing them.

Maedor read the emergence of prayer and meditation as therapeutic
interventions as a "threat" to the Christian understanding of community,
that is, the worship of God and imitation of Christ. He acknowledged
that the religious principle of hospitality from ancient times has been the
ethical and religious rationale of caring for the sick, infirm, and elderly.
But in the current state of medical intervention and application of what
were considered to be devotional principles, that initial understanding
is lost.[66] Once God or Buddha is commodified by transference of devotional practices, the cultural understanding of health is changed, as are
popular perceptions. In addition to changing the economy of media culture, larger psychospiritual changes go on in popular thinking, Maedor
argued, "For once health is made, however implicitly, a product of individual devotional activity, devotion will necessarily be directed toward
the achievement of health. And when devotion is directed toward the
achievement of health, the community's attitude toward the sick and
suffering, toward those who cannot, no matter what they do, become
healthy, will inevitably be changed."[67]

MEDICAL ADVICE AS A COMMODITY

If patients cannot talk to their own doctors, or their spiritual needs are not met by the current medical system, and if they also do not feel as if they belong to any religious denomination, the audience for medial advice in popular books about health embodies a type of "secular" religious language, and the consumer belongs to a pseudo-congregation of popular beliefs based on principles of good health. The history of the medical best seller is inextricably involved with the American religious and literary culture and the search for a healing presence. Since 1975, with the first edition of Herbert Benson's global best-selling *The Relaxation Response*, a spate of best-selling spiritual advice books have held the public attention for weeks on *The New York Times* best-seller list. If Maedor is correct, commodification of spiritual ideas about health have changed how Americans perceive religion and health, and shaped popular ideas about medical and spiritual authority.[68]

As chapter 1 describes, physicians in the late nineteenth century often wrote books of medical advice that became best sellers. Those found in the Rare Book Room of Harvard Medical School's Countway Library—the testimonials, pitch, and hard sell of books about science and religion—are in the tradition of those during the age of hydropathy, mesmerism, mental healing, and homeopathy. They are cultural beauty marks, speaking volumes about how Americans see themselves and what they perceive to be their needs and desires for health.

The advice in these books is studied and practiced, but their advertisements are also instructive about America's search for an instant cure. The advertisements for these books are integrally related, culturally, to the advertisements for drugs; the same Madison Avenue language and mind-set are involved. In Benson's book, *The Relaxation Response*, for example, the concepts are packaged in the language of instant remedy blended with the language of advertising, steeped in the promises of hopes that are usually the province of religion. Reading the language of advertising mixed in with the science and religious ideas illustrates the temper of the late twentieth century, as well as our own times, which Keith Maedor argued we ought to resist, for the good of our souls if not our culture.

In 1975, Benson's agent asked him to write *The Relaxation Response*, according to his own account, which became not only a *New York Times* best seller, but reached global audiences and launched his career, though he still had to do some persuading at Harvard Medical School. Benson probably had nothing to do with the way the book is designed or how it is marketed: his publisher or his agent wrote, "I feel blessed to have discovered the Relaxation Response and subsequently to have realized the power of remembered wellness at a relatively young age. A full third of Americans regularly practice a technique that elicits the Relaxation Response. In 1975, only 7 percent of Americans did so. . . . Today, mind/body techniques and the practice of nourishing one's spirit are mainstream concepts."[69] Whether or not Benson's claim for a "discovery" that actually had been in existence since the beginnings of medical history is overwritten in typical publicity-hype style, the additional claim—that the popularity of Benson's first book prompted the rise of a self-help genre—is justifiable.

Using infomercial language, *The Relaxation Response* promised a panacea for modern life's many stressors "in just minutes a day." Stark was a journalist, assigned to interview him; she became his coauthor later. Benson's research is a cultural map of the 1960s and 1970s: his first applications for the Relaxation Response were in alleviating drug abuse, and early clinical trials included samples among those engaged in transcendental meditation.[70] Benson's is a simple idea based on a "three-legged stool" that includes awareness on the part of the consumer about "self-care, physicians' surgeries and procedures, and pharmacology," and it is good, practical advice based on empirical evidence as well as common sense.

In turning empirical science into a commodity, the agent used advertising and a direct pitch to consumers seeking health. The cover copy for the book's thirtieth anniversary edition is a hard-sell pitch:

> Why this could be the most important book in your life. . . . Sixty to ninety percent of visits to physicians are for conditions related to stress. The Relaxation Response counteracts the harmful effects of stress in a host of conditions including: anxiety, mild and moderate depression, anger and hostility, hypertension, irregular heartbeats,

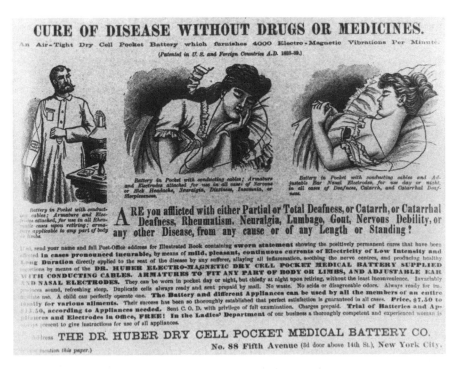

Figure 4.3: *A man and two women each wear a pocket battery pack with connecting cables and electrodes; on the man they are attached to his arm, on the women they are worn around the head and in the ears.* Cure of Disease without Drugs or Medicines. *Newspaper advertisement for battery packs.* Harper's Weekly 33 *(June 15, 1889), 487. Courtesy of the National Library of Medicine.*

pain, premenstrual syndrome, infertility, hot flashes of menopause, insomnia, irritable bowel syndrome, and many other stress-related illnesses. Millions have read about the Relaxation Response in *Time* magazine, *Good Housekeeping*, and *Family Circle* and have seen it described on the *Today* show, *Good Morning America*, and *Nightline*. You can learn simple mind/body techniques to elicit the Relaxation Response without leaving home, and you can use them anywhere. The Relaxation Response is without serious side effects and reaffirms the value of prayer, meditation, and relaxation in your daily life! ... [W]hen Dr. Benson introduced this simple, effective mind/body approach to relieve stress . . . the book became an instant national best seller. Since that time, millions of people have learned the secret of the Relaxation Response—without the high-priced lectures, drugs, or prescription medicine. . . . This revitalizing, therapeutic approach, discovered by Dr. Benson and his colleagues in the laboratories of Harvard Medical School and its teaching hospitals, is now routinely recommended to treat patients suffering from heart conditions, high blood pressure, chronic pain, insomnia and many other physical ailments. Requiring only minutes to learn, and just ten to twenty minutes of practice twice a day, the Relaxation Response has proven to be one of the most effective ways to relieve the tensions of modern-day living for a richer, healthier, more productive life.[71]

Prescribing faith to heal the body through the mind is as controversial today as it was at the beginning of the twentieth century. In America's celebrity culture, where pseudo "doctors" give psychological or spiritual advice on talk shows, many Americans put a magical kind of trust in advice that is "mediated"; that is, science is made simple enough for popular consumption. So those real doctors discussed in this chapter have to persuade their audience about faith as much as they do about hard science.

Chapter 5

THE MEDICATED PUBLIC SQUARE
ADVERTISING SCIENCE

Man is a messenger who forgot the message.

—Abraham Heschel

The American search for a healing presence today occurs in an electronic petri dish where private enterprise and the imagination of disease multiply in symbiotic relationships, creating a climate of hope through pseudo-events and branded promotion. So pervasive is the presence of the pharmaceutical industry in media that the fishbowl transparency caused by twenty-four-hour news where matters of public policy once were debated, called the "Naked Public Square,"[1] has evolved into the "Medicated Public Square," in which the search for a healing presence through streaming, electronic, digital, and photographic images is an outgrowth of the nineteenth century, when toxins were prescribed as heroic cures and suffering in childbirth was considered morally beneficial. Mass media is the central agent in a process of normalizing psychosomatic illness resulting from anxiety: advertising diseases in order to sell the cure forms a contrapuntal refrain to the magical thinking on magazine covers about longevity and the fear of death. The two coexist in an ecology as interdependent as heroic cures and mind cures, the two opposite ends of the healing spectrum that once defined the debate about religion and medicine in the late nineteenth century. Both the desire for the drug panacea as advertised—the instantaneous gratification of a cure for which we can shop—and the longing for eternal life have usurped the blessed assurance once provided by religion and the rational evidence provided by science, making belief into a commodity in a "Medicated Public Square" that makes personal fitness a god while universal health care remains out of reach. This chapter raises questions about the implications of these converged social forces for the broader culture: that is, how does the social economy of medicine fit within a media ecology constructed by political and financial interests working together to create a prescription culture that thrives on fear appeals and anxiety about illness?

Some modern neuroscientists argue that despite advances in medicine, century-old mysteries remain about how psychology and biology interact to create disease. "Medicalizing women," a term that means how Madison Avenue explains the natural physiological stages of aging into a disease, has been a hallmark in the history of American medicine and the drug industry, and in our own postmodern era serves again as the focus of medical media marketing. "Educating consumers" to learn brand names, as children learned the alphabet at the time of the Columbian Exposition, is a marketing method that universalizes psychosomatic illness and links it with mass media fear appeals, which developed during more than a century of promising relief from suffering through medications advertised in a variety of media, from print to the Internet. From the time of the 1893 Chicago Columbian Exposition through 1910, at the time of Rev. Eddy's death, American drug companies created alphabet books for children that educated infants and toddlers about brand names along with their ABCs, as if the language of medication were some sort of catechism. Drug manufacturers in the nineteenth century used beautifully designed trade cards promising cures for many ailments with one compound. Today, the drug industry combines pills that treat high blood pressure with pills that treat high cholesterol, and pills designed to rebuild bone mass have been compounded from once a week to once a month for the consumers' convenience.

Today, when technology is shaping medicine so that doctors are better able to predict, to cure, and to diagnose disease with unprecedented

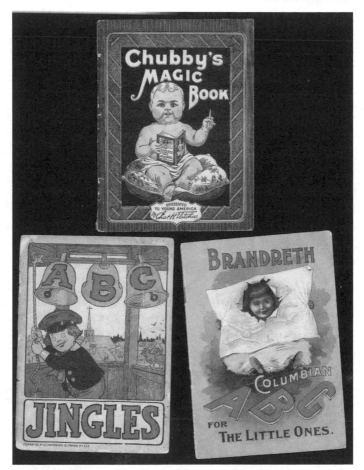

Figure 5.1: Three pharmaceutical advertisement alphabet books. (1)
Chubby's Magic Book, Presented to Young Americans, *by Charles*
H. Fletcher. This was the man who advertised his Castoria stomach
remedy on buildings, ca. 1910. (2) ABC Jingles *(Syracuse, NY: G.C.*
Hanford, 1911). (3) Brandreth Columbian ABC for Little Ones
(New York: Benjamin Brandreth Co., 1893), issued to advertise Allcock's
Porous Plasters, Allcock's Corn and Bunion Shields, and Brandreth's pills.
The latter contains an alphabet of large red capital letters, each illustrated
with scenes in color of Columbus's voyage to America; an illustrated
centerfold of the main buildings at the 1893 Columbian Exposition in
Chicago; and testimonials of eminent persons of cures from using these
products. On the back wrapper is an advertisement for druggist E. R.
Crandall, Winooski, Vermont. The Jane Gilmartin Gilcrest Collection.
Courtesy of the Newberry Library, Wing Collection Foundation.

precision, and when "scientific information" about illness and drugs to alleviate symptoms are offered on the Internet, on television, and in best-selling advice books by celebrity doctors or televangelists, the audience has an unprecedented number of options in multimedia products that deliver a pseudo-religious positivism: "Live your best life now!" While advertising is only one medium among many that disseminate hope as this positivism, it is a highly effective mode, and the most pervasive. The messages that blur medical and spiritual authority—making the American public vulnerable to information about illness created by the drug industry, "nonprofit" consumer and patient groups, global marketing communication firms, lobbying organizations, and a complex of other social forces—shape public policy as well as the climates of personal belief that constitute the "religious" vernacular for those worried about the physical while calling themselves "spiritual."

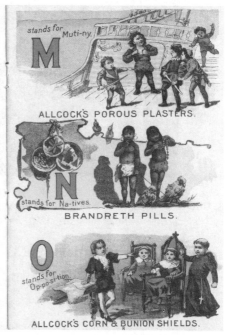

Figure 5.2: Layout of one interior page of one alphabet book with testimonial by famous Americans. Brandreth Columbian ABC for Little Ones *(New York: Benjamin Brandreth Co., 1893). The Jane Gilmartin Gilcrest Collection. Courtesy of the Newberry Library, Wing Collection Foundation.*

We are not in a new era today but one that connects us culturally in values, attitudes, and popular beliefs to our own historical past, within which suffering is misinterpreted, health is misunderstood, and public information or mass education is confused with advertising. The ideas advanced by the complementary and alternative medicine movement about the psychology of fear and faith, and the roles of prayer, belief in healing, and wellness, have been around for well over a century, though the positioning of these ideas in mass media products, particularly best-selling books, touts them as "inventions" of the new age. Yet what is different about the current complementary and alternative medicine movement is the integration of Eastern with Western spirituality.

The Buddhist monk Amaro said recently that in American culture anxiety is a "pandemic," while the scholar Wolinsky wrote that the United States is the global "epicenter" for the innovative use of medicines designed to escape suffering.[2] Americans are 5 percent of the global population but 50 percent of the market for prescription drugs.[3] In the United States, the drug industry is five times more profitable than the oil industry.[4] Only in America and New Zealand is it legal to advertise drugs directly to consumers through television and the Internet, a method so highly effective that thousands of advertisements are submitted annually to the Food and Drug Administration for approval, with the numbers expected to increase. The American Medical Association recently sold information about its 840,000 member physicians to a data bank for pharmaceutical marketing purposes for $44.5 million, raising 16 percent of its annual revenue, according to Big Pharma critics. Researchers in science and in marketing communication have proven that with habits of overmedication, just as in alcohol and tobacco abuse, the child is father to the man. Under U.S. law, testing an existing drug on children can extend a pharmaceutical manufacturer's patent protection. In the first three years of the new millennium, prescribing drugs that medicate the mind to children and adolescents increased by 77 percent, and there was a 50 percent increase in those drugs prescribed for children under five.[5] The impact of this pharmaceutical presence, magnified exponentially through mass media, has created a collective imagination of illness, rather than having advanced a deeper understanding of the spirituality of health, as this chapter asserts.

THE FEAR APPEAL

At the dinner table in many homes in America, there is an unseen presence, a background noise containing messages about health worries. During primetime television newscasts, breaking news often warns audiences about pseudo-epidemics or diseases, such as mercury in dental fillings, a fear appeal on the newscast repeated in advertisements for pharmaceuticals, or unbranded advertising in disease awareness campaigns that generate revenue often echoing the health news of the day. From this convergence between news and advertising, a new vocabulary about health has emerged: conditions no one has heard of previously—restless legs, erectile dysfunction, sleep disorders, female dysphoria, social anxiety disorder, child hyperactivity, aspirin resistance, metabolic syndrome, acid reflux, and child and adult attention deficit disorder—are all "branded" by Madison Avenue. Though these health conditions are not entirely fictitious, they are the work of creative advertising for pharmaceutical corporations; they fit a prescription medication already approved by the Food and Drug Administration for serious illness. When the patent protection for the drug nears expiration, manufacturers hope to extend the patent and protect their profits from generic manufacturers by altering the use of the pill, or its color, name, or dosage, creating a place for its role in alleviating less serious diseases or conditions.[6]

Positioning is not just a matter of medical marketing, but is about changing the spiritual story behind the cultural lens, feeding the collective and individual imagination of consumers about self, health, and disease. So science becomes a mere matter of knowing the shelf life of the message inventory. While in the foreground the unchurched American consumer is just coping with timeless human fears about suffering, illness, or death, in the background is the anxiety-producing drumbeat of medical media marketing in the form of advertising drugs that offer a cure. The moral dilemma here is not merely that popular audiences are fooled by clever messages and are unable to understand medical science, but it is the cultural problem of the trust they put into mass media as a medical and spiritual advisor. Confidence in medical authority has given way to confidence in advertising as an authority: as news stories undermine public confidence in the pharmaceutical industry with stories about lethal side effects of miracle cures, advertising makes promises about healing ailments no one knew they had. Mass media is in the center of this confusion about spiritual authority and scientific evidence with the countercurrents of overclaiming and underreporting, the prosperity of the health communication industry could not exist.

Why do people trust scientific or medical information coming from a television or a computer screen pop-up ad? In part, it is a lack of critical thinking or educated skepticism, based on misinformation about the engineering of medical media marketing. Yet a tendency to believe everything in print is also embedded in our culture, in the ways that the history of American religion and medicine are inextricably intertwined, and in the fused identities of spiritual advisor and medical doctor. In the era when Harvard Medical School was founded, Dr. Walter Channing was often confused with his cousin Rev. William Ellery Channing, in the sense of their social status and spiritual authority. Sophia Peabody and many other Transcendentalists and utopian thinkers relied on the biblical interpretations of both Channings to determine an invalid's proper duties, as future citizens of heaven. When incurable ailments struck, particularly during the childbearing years, women and their husbands followed blindly the directives of both ministers and doctors, both of whom prescribed keeping the faith at the same time they prescribed heroic cures that were experimental, and toxic, and which caused suffering. Though there were malpractice suits enough to warrant a course on medical jurisprudence in the early curriculum of Harvard Medical School, the complete absence of any inclination to blame among those suffering from the experimental cures of early physicians could not have occurred without the spirituality that rationalized suffering.

CULTURAL CONDITIONING

In the twenty-first century a new dimension of faith in medicine and the American cultural search for health and longevity is being constructed through mass media. Magazines from *Newsweek* to *National Geographic* have featured cover stories about "The Search for Health," "The Faith Factor," and "Longevity." When on September 6, 2006, *Time* magazine online released as breaking news a story first carried online weeks earlier by the Public Library of Medicine—the results of a Harvard School of Public Health study about the top seven counties in the United States where life expectancy was greatest—the pop-up advertisement above the *Time* logo online was "Are you taking Lipitor?" This banner headline-size ad hyperlinked with "a clinical study showed that there may be a way to lower your bad cholesterol even further." Journalists pay for media space through advertising revenues, and public interest in the latest stories about religion and health has developed a significant market, one apt to grow as the population ages and longevity increases. The appetite for health and science news about religion and wellness fuels the growth of pharmaceutical advertising. Both news and advertising interests seek audiences, and both need to hold the attention of health-conscious consumers in order to secure ratings and increase revenues.

Are people as concerned about their health and about religion as the current headlines would seem to imply, or is this the veneer of an extensive web of financial interests that link the corporate ownership of global media interests with global pharmaceutical interests and the expertise of advertising and public relations firms with a century of practice as public information and persuasion campaigns? Do the repeated stories in the Medicated Public Square reflect another dimension of social reality: the media ecology that informs the symbiotic relationship between the news side and the advertising side of health in American life today? Admittedly, the ubiquitous advertising messages from the pharmaceutical industry in the twenty-first century are a highly effective, albeit commercial, healing presence. Marketing communication industries transmit sales messages about drugs into the public square through brand advertising and through unbranded information about disease, called awareness campaigns yet termed "information" or "education." While not everyone is taken in by those firms advertising pseudoscience, many people have absorbed new information about medicine through visual images in commercial communication and accepted as authoritative medical advice transmitted through mass media that seemingly describes conditions so universal that they seem to resemble one's own.

When the "remembered wellness" of mind-body medicine is transformed into fears about anticipated illness through mass media industries, the fads and trends in the surface culture slowly create a seismic shift in the deeper culture; in ideas about belief, trust, faith, and hope;

and in the healing power of religion and medicine. We cannot fully understand these changes because we stand in the midst of this mega-trend transforming popular attitudes about health, healing, and belief. This trend is as great as those that mark the historical epochs in the advancement of thinking in medicine in the nineteenth century, when invalids like Sophia Peabody were sent to Cuba after a round of arsenic and mercury, and at the turn of the twentieth century, when evolution, psychology, and the biblically based healing practices of Rev. Eddy emerged from the superstitions that preceded them: water cures and animal magnetism, among others.

Scholars tracing the changes in American religious pluralism tend to look at the rituals and practices where people worship and congregate, but actually, today, ideas about healing in medicine may hold the potential to change religious attitudes, or to indicate how those attitudes are in flux in what has been called a new climate of "medical pluralism" in complementary and alternative medicine. Maybe it is an emerging style of public belief that we have not yet considered instrumental in its power to change social habits and religions.

There is, in the midst of the macronarrative about faith and wellness, an undercurrent of doubt, whether illnesses are real or imagined, whether they exist in the body or are in the mind. If the illnesses are imagined, and certainly advertising relies on the ability of the imagination to connect with stories about a cure, then is the faith that heals merely another demonstration of the placebo effect? What about the power of what contemplative monks and classic mystical literature call the *via negativa*—the void, abyss, emptiness, or dryness of the soul, what doctors interested in the power of faith call the nocebo, the lack of belief in medicine—that diminishes the body's ability to heal?

Doubt results from that constant drumming on the public awareness from the media about things that could happen, whether illness or terrorism, natural catastrophe, or identity theft. The appeal of such news stories based on doubt are rooted in messages about "staying tuned" to alleviate fears, messages designed to retain audiences and improve ratings, and they might very well, cumulatively, contribute to anxiety about illness, especially when coupled with advertising. They also weigh into the psychology of mediated belief. If the threats to health carried in the news could actually happen, based on evidence, then it is not too far a stretch for the imagination to seize on health messages in advertisements that fit in and around the news about diseases that could be contracted, since they are both carried on the same screen. Only purchasing power can assuage this undercurrent of doubt, the retail therapy of shopping, turning medicine into just one among many choices about what to buy. Only control over decisions about products assuage the anxiety caused by the feeling in the audience that an aspect of life is out of their control, that instilled fear is perpetuated by mass media advertising which needs to sell products to validate itself as a revenue stream. Stories in the mass media tend to echo one another, while some of the significant facts are hidden—or as issue managers call it, "sleeping"— in the back pages of the press. But the most revealing facts are often obscured from public consumption—a trend gaining momentum, but in the distance, in the vastness of an electronic ocean, in the current that builds in the momentum of waves that eventually will hit the shore. As market forces build momentum, audiences do not stand still; they move. As attitudes change, so does the big cultural story that is told wherever people assemble and relate a narrative that is biographical, clinical, journalistic, and creatively persuasive in fictitious advertising.

Incredible as it may seem to us in the cold light of day, people actually do believe in the fictional representation of the healing power of medicine in advertisements built on fear appeals. The use of persuasion to convince mass publics that they need medication or the ministrations of doctors for minor ailments to be whole, perfect, and healthy belongs to the tradition of popular belief about health in America, which flourished in the late Victorian era of heroic cures and quackery. How easy it is to look back in time and judge as primitive the heroic quality of the medicine practiced by Dr. Channing and his Harvard contemporaries—how physicians of that day clung to their brutal style of healing. How easy also it is to see as naïve the trust in people's upturned faces, people wearing bowler hats or millinery with ostrich feathers, mere heads in black-and-white photographs now, gathered on the lawn of Rev. Eddy's home and all too ready to forget what they believed in last month. They listened to Rev. Eddy in hopes of being able to witness an ill person being healed through Christ. Thousands of others during the early twentieth century gathered in the South under tents and sang and prayed and thrilled with ecstasy at the laying on of hands. It is the same type of endemic cultural hope that drives the advertising industry today, which uses the figure of a worried middle-aged person—part of what journalists have dubbed the "sandwich generation"—taking care of children and elders at the same time, striking a universal stress point in fears of aging, illness, and physical decline.

In an Aricept advertisement, a worried woman takes care of her children, husband, and father, who has early Alzheimer's. Quick cuts appear of them working in the garden, his forgetfulness extending to how to knot his tie, his willingness to follow her directive that he bring the salad bowl to the dinner table. They are down-home folks with a front-porch swing, Norman Rockwell and the *Saturday Evening Post* people with the postmodern plague of the mind that is to be feared. Inside the house, the woman clicks on her computer screen for a drug Web site, seeking information she needs about the drugs he has been prescribed, while soft music plays in the background and the advertisement on the Web site plays on the television screen. This Aricept advertisement is among the better-crafted, nesting Web site within television advertisement, a voiceover in the woman's own words that the medicine is worth it if it keeps him "normal" for a while longer and able to live at home. The promise of this and other messages like it sell because they connect with the magical thinking behind popular belief in pharmaceutical marketing as scientific information, something that passes for medicine in our own day, which is just as primitive and naïvely wishful and deeply embedded in cultural attitudes that belong historically to the development of medicine in America. This book is about that embedded primitive hope in American religious culture, translated today by complex, subtle, and sometimes altogether hidden interrelationships among government, the drug industry, mass media, doctors, and consumers, all of whom are the workers in today's health information industry.

For most of the twentieth century, those who considered it unethical or illegal to advertise drugs carried the political day, despite congressional debates and the creation of the Food and Drug Administration intended to guard consumers' safety, and the Federal Trade Commission, to guarantee fair competition among drug manufacturers. Only in the last decade of the twentieth century did the U.S. Congress legalize direct-to-consumer (DTC) drug advertising.[7] Only U.S. policymakers miss the connection between public information about health, a marketing pitch for prescription drugs, and the "invention" of imaginary illness or "disease mongering."[8]

MENTAL CONDITIONING

Consider that clinical trials funded by pharmaceutical companies conclude, based on scientific research, that some class of drug cures a particular disease. This is announced in a press release by a nonprofit disease association and picked up by journalists as news of a cure. Maybe the TV station's physician (M.D.), who serves as their medical science reporter, comments in a two-minute package on the half-hour evening primetime newscast, one-quarter of which is devoted to pharmaceutical advertising. This news information from press releases is followed by advertisements for a patented drug of that same type, or what is called unbranded disease awareness advertising.[9] In order to develop a niche market, the definition of a branded condition is expanded to include increasing numbers of people who do not "yet have" any disease, especially children and healthy adults with minor ailments. Conflicts of interest among physicians with ties that are too close to the drug industry abound, as critics have observed. Though some doctors argue that advertising drugs creates the emotional conditioning that will enhance the placebo effect when the medication is taken, resistance to the culture of Big Pharma is manifested in a variety of new beliefs and hopes about longevity and a healing presence.[10] In part, that resistance has contributed to the burgeoning consumer-driven complementary and alternative medicine movement, as chapters 3 and 4 outline.

CAM asserts that the human body thrives when the natural harmony of internal neurological balance is maintained through calm emotions. This occurs when the mind is at peace, in sync with its environment, well nourished, reaching up to Divine Wisdom or God, and reaching out to others. This spiritual understanding of health advocates not only balance but also a realization of impermanence, in the Buddhist context, and an understanding of "counting our days aright," in the Psalmist's language. There is value in simply being, more than in being busy, in a culture of overproductive children, workers, and parents, and a value in mind training that develops concentration, the threshold of awareness. Some prescribe "media fasting," so great is the estimated impact of 24/7 connectivity in a wireless and virtual universe.[11] In the CAM lexicon, negative emotions are toxic—and none more so than anger, fear, or anxiety. Both precipitate the stress response that disrupts the internal biochemical balance within a healthy body, causing disease. Within that context, prayer and meditation are regarded as therapeutic interventions.

Saturating the media with messages and branding new disease conditions alters what should be the balance of trust between patient and health care provider. Patients who see or read advertisements for drugs initiate the process of prescription. Drugs are not the same as other products, as Big Pharma critics point out.[12] They cost far more, for one thing, and taking them can change an individual's self-perception from someone who is healthy and well, to someone who identifies with their disease. As a cultural habit in an economy of consumption, drugs have an impact on ideology as well as theology; the prescription culture alters ideas of medical and spiritual authority and has an impact on the broader political order in terms of public policy and what is considered ethically acceptable.

MARKETPLACE CONDITIONING

As drugs go through three clinical phases of testing, from discovery to approval to the marketplace, a parallel promotional mechanism prepares the marketplace for consumption of the pill when it does reach the market. This decade-long strategic planning occurs incrementally:

1. The market is identified by manufacturers.
2. New uses for existing prescriptions are linked with the disease or conditions.
3. A disease or patient Association is formed, with support from the pharmaceutical industry, which establishes a data bank of those with the disease or whose family members have the disease.
4. That Association launches multimedia products, including a Web site, newsletter, bulletins about development, a magazine, and regional special events to raise funds and visibility of the Association.

5. The Association sponsors research about itself, publishing the results of polls and surveys as well as scientific research in its publications and press releases.

6. The medical journalist picks up from the press release the "story" behind the cure for a disease.

7. A celebrity champion emerges who either has the disease or says they have had a family member with the disease.

8. Momentum picks up when word makes its way into the Medicated Public Square, and lobbyists are hired, targeting federal regulatory or elected officials, resulting in a legal climate conducive to sales.

By the time a drug is submitted for approval, the promotional campaign has been planned. The advertising agency can step in, prepare direct-to-consumer advertisements that tell the general population who are not ill to "ask their doctor" about a specific prescription. When the drug is approved by the FDA and medical liaisons are ready to talk with doctors, giving out free samples, the consumer is also ready to listen to the advertising, go to the Web site, and print out information, and then ask the doctor for the medicine while it is at peak cost, under patent. The other psychosocial effects in this decade-long process are more nuanced and subtle. As the Association forms, people who do have the disease begin to think about their identity associatively, with others who also belong to an affinity group, people similarly identified by either having or knowing someone with a specific set of afflictions. Identifying with a group both reinforces the identification between patients and their malady, and legitimates their symptoms by connecting them with a larger public. As a drug is developed, champions cluster, and special events involving legislators and celebrities draw more media attention.

The struggle for getting, keeping, and extending patent protection drives a process that costs twice as much as scientific research and development. Lobbyists speed up the approval process of new drugs by the FDA, and extend the companies' holds on original patents and the "exclusive marketing rights" granted by the FDA, as Angell described.[13] This image of what critics call Big Pharma, the Pharmaceutical Research and Manufacturing Association or PhRMA, is contested by the industry itself through counterclaims based on the cost of research and development, though the National Institutes of Health funded by taxpayers is respon-sible for much of the research.

REGULATORY CONDITIONS

PhRMA's annual report asserts that the costs of producing life-saving medications are justified: it takes $800 million and ten to fifteen years on average to discover, test, and approve one new drug. Pharma critics argue that much of the groundbreaking research is farmed out to uni-versity scientists and NIH, already funded by U.S. taxpayers, so those cost estimates are inflated. The industry reports that only five in five thousand compounds make it into the phase of human testing, and of those, only one is approved, on average.[14]

The three phases of discover, test, and approve are as laborious as they are costly. In the initial discovery process, drugs are tested on labo-ratory animals for about six or seven years. In Phase II clinical trials lasting about two years test the drug on progressively larger human pop-ulations for progressively longer periods. Initially, twenty to one hundred healthy volunteers test the drugs for eighteen months to discern dosage and safety. Sometimes prisoners are used, which is a highly controversial practice. Then groups of one hundred to five hundred patient volunteers evaluate the effectiveness of the drug and look for side effects. Phase III lasts for three to four years, testing the drug on one thousand to five thou-sand patient volunteers to confirm effectiveness, and to monitor adverse reactions from long-term use. At this point, the application for approval goes to the FDA, containing all the information from the testing period: applications typically exceed one hundred thousand pages. The average review time for the thirty-six new therapeutic drugs approved by the FDA in 2004 was about a year and a half. During that review process, "pre-launch" publicity prepares consumers for the medicine when it is available, though PhRMA's "guiding principles" for direct-to-consumer advertising effective in early 2006 argue that all companies should not only submit the ads to the FDA but also wait for their approval before releasing them for broadcast. DTC brand ads should clearly state the health condition and risks associated with the medication, present a bal-anced view of the risks versus the benefits, and present visuals that do not distract viewers from absorbing the information; also, companies should spend "an appropriate amount of time" educating health professionals with "valid" information about a new medicine obtained "from reliable sources," prior to launching a DTC campaign.[15]

Once approved and under patent, manufacturers have a narrow time frame within which to recover costs before patents expire and the FDA permits lower-cost generics to compete. Once a company loses patent rights, sales of the higher-cost drug drop; any pharmacist can fill a prescription with the cheaper generic unless the prescribing physician specifies a brand. Angell cited Roger Williams of the FDA, who said, "There are anywhere from ten to twenty tactics" used by the drug industry to "protect" their brand, including changing pill color, dose, or name. For example, "new molecular entities" may justify a five-year patent; "orphan drugs" (those with an expected market of less than two hundred thousand) may receive seven years, and three years for changes in already approved drugs: "The anti-generic strategy by pharmaceutical companies has probably the highest rate of return of any business activity they do right now," Angell has charged.[16] Since the trial period can last ten to fifteen years, many patents could be as brief as five years, unless the corporation can invent new uses.

Among the chief legislative benchmarks in the drug economy are the 1984 Hatch-Waxman Act, which increased generic sales by 30 percent; FDA-updated patent limits from seventeen to twenty years in 1994; and in 1997, the FDA "Modernization Act" extended patent protection for an additional six months if the new drugs were tested on children.[17]

The future of pharmaceuticals, in the words of the industry, are toward "targeted personalized medicines" to improve treatment and reduce side effects, based on how genetic traits influence how people respond to medicines.[18] Personalized medicine based on genetics, with customized marketing and the broad global reach through mass media in direct-to-consumer advertising, as part of large-scale disease awareness campaigns combine to create a powerful influence in American culture. Potentially, this personalization, customization, and mass marketing can shape how people see themselves, how medical practitioners treat people who are sick, and how influential government elites think about the national health care infrastructure, in financial, political, and spiritual terms.

OLD PILLS IN NEW CAPSULES

Financial pressure on the manufacturer to find multiple uses for drugs already approved in order to extend a patent and the period when the drug pulls in the greatest profit margin creates the market within which manufacturers and marketers brand conditions as diseases. The most famous of these was Viagra, originally intended for heart patients with angina, its sexual side-effect repositioned the drug as a market leader. Schering-Plough's lucrative allergy pill Claritin became Clarinex, and the Prozac associated with negative publicity and the stigma of mental illness was called Sarafem. Requip is a compound that regulates the dopamine levels in the brain, developed from an off-label use of a drug developed to treat Parkinson's.[19]

Recently, Woloshin and Schwartz quantified how journalists are complicit in this marketing process by not probing deeply enough into press releases about science. The two academics tracked through content analysis how news reports disseminated stories about the new disease, "Restless Leg Syndrome" (RLS), an "urge to move the legs" occurring mainly at night, invented by GlaxoSmithKline in order to market Requip.[20] Echoing arguments made earlier by Payer, Parry, Moynihan, and Cassels, the coauthors used content analysis of news media to document how journalists aid and abet the phenomenon. The consumer population for the product is brought about by lowering the threshold levels that define the disease and by normalizing the condition through advertising.

Jeanne Whalen, a journalist for the *Wall Street Journal*, later picked up and repeated the story of how Requip's sales reached $500 million a year less than four years after the disease was invented by the pharmaceutical manufacturer, following a television advertising campaign selling the disease. The journalist summarized the evidence about the drug without mentioning that the pharmaceutical firm that invented the disease had any connection with the RLS Foundation consulted by journalists as the "expert medical authority" that legitimated the disease, an organization that she cited in the concluding paragraph of her article. As Whalen told the story, the disease invention occurred in three phases: first, by advertising in medical journals to doctors, employing a doctor to give dozens of talks about the subject; then, after about two years, spending $36 million on television advertising, which doubled the number of "hits" on the RLS Foundation Web site to 4,500 per day within two months of the advertising campaign launch: "Less than half of Requip's expected $500 million in sales are expected to come from Parkinson's disease; the rest should come from RLS, a Citigroup Inc. research report estimates."[21]

Woloshin and Schwartz deconstructed how journalists helped disseminate the RLS disease by responding uncritically to promotional messages early on, and they concluded based on their research results that journalists lack the skepticism necessary to do their jobs in reporting on medicine.[22] This may be too sweeping a generalization based on evidence from one case study and might be unfair to journalists to some degree, yet by studying news reports such as the one cited above from the *Wall Street Journal*, their conclusions about the superficiality of reporting on the pharmaceutical industry seems to hold up. Woloshin and Schwartz's work also may demonstrate that many journalists, though well intentioned, do not know enough about the advertising and public relations industry that the pharmaceutical manufacturers use to generate "news": journalists report "on faith" what they hear from the industry, without looking deeply enough into how the promotional side of the news industry creates a need for a product with too small a market and too great a research investment. In any event, the invention of the disease contributes to a climate of distrust for the pharmaceutical industry among the consumers that seems to be in advance of the journalists. Yet one network has begun to involve pharmaceutical corporations as "sponsors" of segments such as NBC's "What Works," in addition to advertising.

Woloshin and Schwartz conducted an analysis of press stories written in response to the press release announcing GSK's presentation of the syndrome to the American Academy of Neurology's annual meeting in 2003. At this meeting, GSK reported on Phase II trials of the drug Ropinirole, a drug first approved for use in Parkinson's disease. The "invention" of the Restless Leg Syndrome that deprives an individual of sleep also develops the prior market for sleep disorders; by linking the two, the industry is giving the impression that one discovery is linked with another in an ongoing meta-story about the social costs of exhaustion and sleep deprivation in lower productivity and highway safety. But this is my speculation, not found in the journalists' coverage.

Woloshin and Schwartz studied 187 articles containing the phrase "restless legs." They found that only one article questioned the disease definition, none questioned the GSK estimate, and two-thirds repeated without questioning that "12 million Americans suffer with it," merely adopting the language of the news release. Three-quarters of the news articles emphasized the social cost of the new disease, 40 percent supplementing the contention with anecdotes, none of which were about those who had RLS but those who were not bothered by it. One-fifth of the articles referred readers to the "nonprofit" Restless Leg Foundation, but none of those included the support of GSK for the foundation. One-third of articles used "miracle language" to describe patient response to medication, while the results of the clinical trial show only about 22 percent difference between those who took the placebo and those who took the drug. Only five of the fifteen articles noted side effects of nausea or dizziness; and only one wrote three years was too short a clinical trial for a drug that would be prescribed for lifetime use. The academic coauthors concluded that "the media seemed to have been co-opted into the disease-mongering process."[23]

A comparable example, drawn from the trade press, is the zeal for invention expressed in an article by Breitstein in *Pharmaceutical Executive* magazine, detailing the launch of the disease called "Metabolic Syndrome," or insulin resistance.[24] Dubbed the "Deadly Quartet," physicians long have known the connection between high cholesterol, hypertension, and impaired glucose tolerance levels could lead to diabetes and cardiovascular disease. In 2001 the National Cholesterol Education Program was a "call to action" for physicians, published in the *Journal of the American Medical Association* that lowered the pre-disease levels of cholesterol, blood pressure, and related biochemistry. Metabolic Syndrome then received its own code in the International Classification of Diseases, Ninth Revision, when it "crossed an important threshold," according to the author, "as an actual disease state."[25]

After that, Breitstein reported, "Pharma opened its floodgates and began to publicly fund market development initiatives to make physicians more aware of the role of insulin resistance in diabetes and heart disease." "The pace of development is accelerating," she wrote, and reported that insulin resistance as a disease emerged from a collaboration between the American College of Cardiology and the American Diabetes Association, resulting in a "making the link" public information campaign to educate physicians and consumers about the connection between Type 2 diabetes, heart disease, and stroke.[26] MSAToday .com, the syndrome's Web site, linked with a "corresponding Web site funded by unrestricted grants from GlaxoSmith-Kline" offering physicians information and continuing medical education credit. The first annual meeting about the disease was followed early the following year with a new society, the International Society of Diabetes and Vascular Research, which published its own journal. Just as the "emergence of cholesterol reduction as a market was a major event" for the industry, the invention of Metabolic Syndrome "promises to be as big or bigger."

Breitstein reported to industry members that "it's not just that metabolic syndrome has become better understood, better publicized, or better supported by an infrastructure of journal articles, meetings, and associations. Behind those events and dozens more like them something far more basic is happening: A new disease is being born. Unlike a new pathogen bursting from the jungle like Ebola or mutating from something familiar like each year's 'new' strain of influenza, metabolic syndrome must be both socially and scientifically constructed." In the short space of six years, "communications about the new disease have reached a critical mass," the author reported, with an abundance of articles in journals and plentiful Web sites supported by drug companies containing information that the "average mindful physician should have heard about," Richard Nesto of Harvard was quoted as having said.[27]

As levels of the predisease states are lowered, PhRMA's estimates for the potential market for the drug expands, and the statistics defining "normal" fit neatly into fear appeals in advertising and in the cautionary "news you can use" tone of multimedia news that compel audiences to "stay tuned." The "obesity epidemic" based on industry estimates of 20 percent of the American public as obese, a number expected to "climb to 40 percent" over the next decade. PhRMA cited the NIH statistic that an American born in 2000 has a one in three chance of developing diabetes, and the American College of Cardiology estimated that prevalence of heart disease will double by 2040.[28] The PhRMA reporter used this evidence to announce the industry estimate that "86 million Americans will have metabolic syndrome by 2025." This leaves the industry to develop compound medications so that the population at risk is not left with a "cocktail of therapies," according to industry reports.[29]

"Pharma companies are running for this market," one pharmaceutical manager is reported as having said. But in the midst of opportunity, the author concludes, "finding pharma's niche in a massive, prevention-oriented campaign . . . won't be easy." The forecasters in the industry are looking at "the 35-year-old office workers who do not get enough exercise or eat right" as their future moneymaker. Not everyone who is overweight shows the symptoms of the syndrome, but Pharma realizes that lifestyle can cure the condition.[30]

IN "PR" WE TRUST

Leading communication experts who advise pharmaceutical executives, such as Lynn Vos, CEO of Grey Healthcare, a former nurse and pharmaceutical executive, acknowledged that the American public's lack of trust in the medical establishment is a direct result of how the public perceives the drug industry. Most recently, pharmaceutical firms have aired image ads with their CEO as a spokesperson, repositioning their reputations by claiming trustworthy achievements through civic concern. But those in the business of reputation management know that advertisements are useful after a product has been positioned in the marketplace through public relations, but if there is already a lack of public trust in a product or company, advertising exacerbates that suspicion. According to one publicity firm, "Advertising has no credibility with consumers, because the public has been increasingly skeptical of its claims and whenever possible are inclined to reject its messages."[31]

The many legal challenges to the advertising claims of the drug industry over the past decade have steadily eroded public trust. Recent lawsuits against Merck for the drug Vioxx allegedly raised the incidence of heart attacks. Legal suits have been resolved on two sides—a $51 million verdict in New Orleans, which may be reversed on appeal as this book is being published; a $253.4 million verdict to a widow in Texas; and a $13.5 million verdict in New Jersey.[32] The cancer drug

Raloxifene, intended to prevent breast cancer, allegedly raised the danger of blood clots and strokes.[33] Fosamax, designed for women with bone-thinning osteoporosis, has been linked in news stories to death of the areas of the jawbone, or osteonecrosis. The FDA also curbed prescriptions for Accutane, an acne drug that caused serious birth defects, liver damage, and suicidal thoughts.[34] Other types of headlines have contributed to a drop in investor confidence, such as when FBI agents raided offices at Bristol-Myers to obtain paperwork to prosecute the company over accusations that they and Sanofi-Aventis offered $40 million to Apotex, Inc., of Canada to delay its marketing of a generic version of Plavix until 2011, when its patent protection expired.[35] The cholesterol reduction drug Lipitor, produced by Pfizer, termed a "blockbuster," allegedly caused memory loss and severe nerve damage and changed behavior among 110,000 of the 22 million who currently take the drug.[36]

Yet some promotion professionals point out that the existing lack of trust among many because of the failure to "educate" has precipitated more subtle methods of marketing through public relations campaigns. Vos advised clients to follow the rubric, "When self-promotion goes up, your opportunity for trust goes down."[37]

Grey Healthcare Group leads the pack among global firms with expertise in reputation management and crisis communication, including other global communication firms such as Omnicom, Interpublic, Edelman, Ruder Finn, Chicco Agency, Medical Action Communications, Shire Health Group, and Meditech Media (UK).[38] Grey is a global company with annual billings of more than $1 billion and with 725 employees in forty-two offices in twenty-one countries— three times the reach it had ten years ago. Grey promotes what it calls its "innovative" ideas about "educating" patients and physicians from a full-service agency with traditional expertise in advertising, public relations, medical education, direct marketing, and market research as well as campaign design. "Pharmaceutical marketing used to be a sacred industry," Vos said in an industry publication interview after receiving a Woman of the Year award from the Healthcare Businesswoman's Association.[39] "At a time when trust in pharma is falling and the public increasingly sees marketing as just another word for manipulation, seemingly everyone is all too aware that there is marketing to doctors, and now to consumers—and all too eager to put an end to it."[40]

In order to rebuild public confidence in the pharmaceutical industry, health care public relations experts like Vos advise exchanging "detailing" for "intimacy" as a marketing communications strategy. Detailing refers to printed materials that are data intensive, such as disease kits, backgrounders with scientific information, and perhaps publications in medical journals or other targeted publications. Intimacy is a one-on-one approach, using trained liaisons culled from the more than eighty thousand sales representatives currently working in the pharmaceutical industry. Vos said in an interview with the trade publication *Pharmaceutical Executive* that "intimacy means that you have to understand the doctor—where they live, what their issues are, how we can help them effect a better practice."[41]

This comment is interesting on two counts: from a strategic positioning standpoint and from the cultural standpoint that a global advertising and public relations firm is taking a reactive role to counter the CAM movement by "reinventing" how doctors practice medicine by altering their understanding of patients from cases to consumers. Vos said, "We've got to get the trust back," and in order to do so she suggests, "let's not just present them with data. Let's present them with some interesting consumer insights. We know about consumers . . . let's actually help them be more effective physicians. Let's improve their credibility."[42]

When Madison Avenue first took on consumer advertising of drugs after 1997, Vos explained, communication experts "agonized" over "how to explain" to doctors the "contradictory messages" in the public square about the " safety of certain medicines." For example, when one Pharma "watchdog" drew up a "list of dangerous drugs he wanted taken off the market," and "four out of five" were Grey clients, the communication people were put on the defensive.[43] Central to their thinking in designing reactive campaigns were key questions relevant to doctors as a demographic cohort: What do doctors think when they pick up their morning newspaper and read headlines about the lethal side effects of prescription medicine? Who can blame them for flinching, knowing that the drugs they might have prescribed are being targeted by watchdogs and perhaps thinking about the cost of malpractice lawsuits?

With direct-to-consumer advertising legal, the goal is to create a new type of brand awareness among medical consumers. Vos said, "Today, when patients show up at the physicians' offices armed with Internet pages on their conditions, and sometimes strong opinions on how they should be treated, a simple warning isn't enough. There is a real need for material that helps physicians do their jobs. We need to arm them with better understanding of the consumer, of what's going on in patients' minds so they can practice better medicine." In global agencies, communication professionals like Vos are trying to build into the physician's clinical habits new ways of thinking about prescribing. At Pfizer, where she had been a top executive, Vos had coined the term "interactive medicine" to help doctors communicate with patients. This approach has been replaced with a new, interactive Web-based schema, "The Doctor Will Hear You Now," an attempt to "get the doctor and the patient on the same page, so doctors will better understand the insights of consumers." Along with cultivating better communication between doctor and patient-consumer, Vos champions full disclosure as a way of rebuilding trust. "Doctors like full disclosure," she said. "It gives them a greater comfort level."[44]

In another article from *Pharmaceutical Executive*, Don Apruzzese, director of marketing for Astra Zeneca, received the industry's PhAME award for an upbeat, nonbranded advertisement that featured survivors of breast cancer "educating" other women about how to avoid reoccurrence. He argued that education rather than branding was the more effective strategy, especially when such an emotionally charged disease as breast cancer "has a palette of colors" associated with it. He argued that his company did the right thing to use an unbranded campaign, so that it would not be seen as "taking advantage of an emotional situation." He forecast more unbranded advertising in the future, with sufficient emotion in the images and script to "drive viewers to other places," including the Web, telephone, and their physician in order to obtain further information.[45]

The tendency toward education rather than branded advertising is driven by the drug safety fiascos responsible for the lack of public trust, such as hormone replacement therapy (HRT). Mintzes observed that in marketing of HRT, menopause was positioned in terms of "increased health risk."[46] Though this observation is astute, it should be considered in historical context with the experiences of women in the nineteenth century.

The progress of American medicine since the founding of Harvard has advanced in knowledge and in profitability by "medicalizing" female physiology, and today that tendency to medicate what once was called female hysteria or neurasthenia is now repackaged in postpartum depression, PMS, and female dysphoria. Another all too transparent ploy, the invention of "female sexual dysfunction," the female equivalent of "erectile dysfunction," was rolled out just after the blockbuster sales of Viagra. Older females could now be cured of a waning libido by wearing a testosterone patch modeled on the nicotine patch to help people quit smoking. The marketing logic here has a kind of satiric beauty: if older men were to consume more Viagra, they would need interested partners. Older women would be brought into the consumer package by reinforcing their "romantic" quotient, reinforcing their self-esteem by implying they, too, might now outgrow the Madison Avenue clichés about sex appeal.

In the continuing saga, Merck turned around and marketed an estrogen patch to reverse a so-called estrogen deficiency. This PR language, at least to my ears, reverberates as the ghost voice of Walter Channing's contemporaries writing letters to him about women's nature in his etherization tract, or his letter to Sophia about how her mind was like any other limb that, when long disused, would atrophy. In our postmodern era, a Web site declaring that women of a certain age with the tendency toward a lower estrogen level can expect "reduced performance," including "fine motor skills, memory," and an alleged inability to engage in "planned, targeted, flexible and adaptable thought," is rooted lock, stock, and barrel into the type of mind-set that framed the life of the neurasthenic a century ago, and "medicalized" the female from childbirth to old age.[47] Wyeth Pharmaceuticals, another company involved in estrogen marketing, created "The Journalist's Menopause Handbook," apparently one that did not include any mention of the side effects of increased risk of stroke, heart attacks, pulmonary emboli, or dementia associated with use of hormonal replacement therapy, according to the critics of Big Pharma.[48] A savvy female communication executive like Vos demonstrated her expertise in managing crises well after the rollout for the HRT drug Premarin, which contained estrogen drawn from horse urine and was widely prescribed and used before the negative publicity over allegations that it caused many deaths diminished its popularity. After the backlash against the drug, Wyeth "repositioned" it "with full disclosure," an antidote to public fears, listing side effects "if used for a long time" and recommending "short-term use, taking as little as possible," strategic PR that revived the market for the drug.[49]

CRITICS OF BIG PHARMA

"There is an unseen presence in the doctor's office," according to critics who interpret the education outreach of health communication professionals to be part of an adverse conditioning of the American consumer. But even among those most critical of Big Pharma, they admit that advances in pharmacology have saved lives, and that the miracle drugs that heal and cure are significant scientific achievements in modern pharmacology.[50] Indeed, it is not the purpose of this book to argue against drugs or the achievements of medicines that have accomplished so much. Like many people who take care of their elders, I have seen firsthand in a cancer ward the "chain of life" where each "link" is a success story, and though drugs save lives every day, disease is the great leveler, without regard for age, creed, or skin color.

Yet it is the mediated veneer of the cure and the huckster quality of drug advertising that evoke the late Victorian era of quackery. The headlines about drug safety violations and harmful death lawsuits in the press are reminiscent of an earlier era, the age of heroic cures in the nineteenth century that experimented with mercury, arsenic, and ether on compliant, vulnerable patients. Advertising and marketing campaigns contribute to a cultural climate of distrust for medical science, and, as I have asserted earlier, history demonstrates that there is an inverse relationship between trust in medical authority and spiritual authority. When people fail to trust doctors, they turn to alternatives that include spiritual advice about how to cope with disease, disappointment, and fear of illness. Often, the media is the alternative authority.

For all the sophistication of modern medicine, things have not advanced far enough, because the complex forces of mass media, electoral politics, public relations, and lobbying work together so well that the pharmaceutical industry is the most profitable sector on Wall Street— despite the lack of public trust. For all the refinement of technology applied to medicine, according to the Institute of Medicine's most recent report, medication errors cost the taxpayer an estimated $3.5 billion annually, harm 1.5 million people, and are responsible for 98,000 deaths.[51]

Critser, Angell, Moynihan, Casssels, and Law, all experts in their respective areas of medical journalism, each with more than two decades of experience, have written recent trade books analyzing the current state of the prescription culture at the beginning of the twenty-first century. Law, a British journalist for *Scrip*, a pharmaceutical journal, wrote an exposé of the global nature of the Vioxx and antidepressant scandals. Moynihan and Cassels dissected how ordinary, moderate health risks have been turned into illness by conflict-of-interest among doctors whose ties are too close to pharmaceutical manufacturers. Angell charged that doctors are complicit in the monopolistic economy of the pharmaceutical industry, and she made mincemeat of Big Pharma's defense for the high cost of drugs. While the Pharma claim is that high costs result from research and development, those costs are only half of the amount spent on advertising, marketing, and direct sales to consumers through doctors, as Angell charged. Crister used basic marketing theory and Maslowe's categories segmenting the population according to their psychological needs to construct a psychographic to analyze the artifice that blurs media marketing and health education.[52]

Crister sorted Americans into three GenRx tribal groups: High-Performance Youth, Middle Years, and Superseniors.[53] The first is the tribe of overprescription, of Ritalin and attention deficit hyperactivity disorder, including approximately five million children and adolescents.[54] Further, as one *New York Times* reporter pointed out, as this tribe matures, in their twenties and thirties, they self-medicate, trading prescriptions with friends and peers, including stimulants, antidepressants and other psychiatric medications.[55] Crister reported that well over half of all youth in the United States are taking at least one antidepressant, a fact responsible for the 77 percent increase between 2000 and 2003: "For the first time, drugs for childhood and adolescent mental health problems pulled ahead of antibiotics and asthma meds, the traditional market dominators in that age group."[56]

Meanwhile, their parents and grandparents, GenRx2, concerned about cholesterol, blood pressure, and blood sugar, are "a tribe of conscious risk dodgers," as well as those with adult ADD, and the sleepless (Ambien) and groggy (Cephalon).[57] Gastrointestinal medications for this tribe are another enormous market—for heartburn, "acid reflux," and a number of pills developed for branded conditions.

Moynihan and Cassels charge that, in the marketing of "lifestyle" drugs (those pills that might be eliminated by changes in lifestyle), there are conflicts of interest among physicians that exponentially widen the market for predisease states.[58] Crister and others go so far as to suggest that by lowering the "minimals," the market soon will include nearly everyone in the nation who has celebrated their fiftieth birthday.[59] Between 1990 and 2001, according to Moynihan, when National Institutes of Health guidelines for cholesterol were set and five of the fifteen authors had financial ties to statin manufacturers, the norms included an additional 23 million more Americans. Three years later, another 40 million more were added when the guidelines were revised by a committee on which eight of the nine authors had financial ties to drug companies, serving as "paid speakers, consultants or researchers" to Pfizer, Merck, Bristol-Myers Squibb, Novartis, Bayer, Abbott, AstraZeneca, and GlaxoSmithKline.[60] Some had ties to more than one drug company; one expert had ties to ten, none of which were acknowledged when the guidelines were published until Reuters broke the news.[61]

GenRx3 are Superseniors—those who are more active, live longer, and a prime market for drugs for joint ailments, pain, memory, and the libido—and the frail elderly. Crister alleges that in long-term care homes, 58 percent of residents are on some form of medication for behavior management.[62]

Yet for all the solid evidence cited in these books by Pharma critics, the ethical questions embedded in marketing communication in health care never quite make it into the news. Marketing drugs to physicians is a $12-billion-a-year industry that spends about $8,000 to $15,000 annually *per physician* in the United States, employing one sales representative for every five physicians.[63] The infantry of "sales representatives" who legally cannot discuss off-label uses of pills have been upgraded to "medical liaisons," a higher rank of the sales function requiring more education and specialized training. Legally, they can talk with doctors about the pill's "off-label" uses and even sit in on patient consultations in some cases.[64] "One's physician may well be a paid pharmaceutical thought leader, getting $10,000 a pop for speeches to his fellows in which he or she talks up a new medication . . . getting paid for 'case studies'—in essence a copy of your experience . . . after you try the new drug."[65] As the evidence builds, doubts deepen, and trust decreases.

Between 1997 and 2002, when restrictions on direct-to-consumer advertising eased, the drug industry ads linked psychographics with emotional pitches through lifestyle marketing; that is, using images because they epitomized a profile of a typical consumer by age, race, and demographics.[66] As Moynihan and Cassels described, selling drugs to people who are ill is one thing, but the net effect of the growth, prevalence, and dominance of the pharmaceutical industry in direct-to-consumer advertising is to universalize the disease state, "aggressively" targeting "the healthy and the well," selling to everybody. The people and faces featured in drug advertising are presented as normal, in control of their lives, mentally strong, upper middle class, upwardly mobile, educated, but "no match for what is about to hit them," as the Plavix anti-clot medication ad phrased it. Moynihan described the ethos:

> The ups and downs of daily life have become mental disorders, common complaints are transformed into frightening conditions, and more and more ordinary people are turned into patients. With promotional campaigns that exploit our deepest fears of death, decay, and disease, the $500 billion pharmaceutical industry is literally changing what it means to be human. . . . At a time when many of us are leading longer, healthier, and more vital lives than our ancestors, saturation advertising and slick 'awareness raising' campaigns are turning the worried well into the worried sick."[67]

The shift from image to awareness, from broad to narrow, cast toward an increasingly customized marketing approach, may speed the approval process or connect with consumers in ways that are more "intimate" and less "detailed," to borrow Vos's strategic marketing vocabulary—but the net effect undermines public trust in science while building hopes through advertising.

One way health care public relations cultivates intimacy with consumers is through patient advocacy groups, building a collective identity based on a shared association with disease, a tremendous data bank of people who are good targets for cause-related marketing campaigns. Knowing the tendency of a cohort to identify as belongers to disease groups is a tremendous resource for sales. They are typically highly interconnected with one another, linked with other patient groups. Externally, their publicity for the profile of the disease and their existence as "nonprofit" organizations legitimate the condition and serve as a resource for mass media, which need information to announce the "discovery," including celebrities or others who have the syndrome, and polls, surveys, or other data about trials and cures. Patient organizations typically publish newsletters, publicize the results of studies, and help "build credibility" because patient advocacy groups are not linked in the public mind with advertising and are perceived to be unbiased; however, these groups are also funded by pharmaceutical companies.[68] For example, Children and Adults with Attention-Deficit Hyperactivity Disorder Association receives one-fifth of its total budget of about $3 million from drug companies.[69]

ADD seems to be widespread yet little understood, not unlike nervous disorders and hysteria, the pervasive malaise of the nineteenth century that afflicted so many, from Sophia Peabody to Charles Darwin. N. W. Read pointed out that "hysteria is no longer considered acceptable" as a term, but the psychosomatic illnesses to which it once referred are still valid. We hear it in contemporary newspeak, and it has turned up in illnesses such as Gulf War Syndrome, Chronic Fatigue Syndrome, Alien Abduction Syndrome, eating disorders, and childhood asthma, all cultural expressions of "intolerable emotional tension."[70] Scientific research results contest the extent to which ADD is a disease of the imagination as well as the mind. Research in scientific journals demonstrates that ADD is a biological disorder, but an equal number of solid investigations by scientists in journals conclude that the condition is not biologically defined; there is no reliable test for it beyond prescribing drugs and waiting to see if they ameliorate symptoms, "and little proof that ADD is a neurological disease," in Moynihan's opinion.[71] While the idea is persuasive that ADD "hyperactivity" is caused by cultural and social factors, the more significant fact is the extent to which the prescription to cure the epidemic is based on contested scientific evidence. The cause of ADD is as mysterious a childhood epidemic as austism, allegedly linked to the mercury in childhood vaccinations.[72] However, both the drug manufacturers and the patient groups describe ADD as a "neurobiological disorder," with very few journalists investigating the dispute behind the claim. Moynihan's figures are shocking: In the six years between 1996 and 2002, sales of the ADD drug Adderall surged $510 million.[73] Between 2000 and 2003, the market for ADD drugs *for children under five* increased 50 percent.[74] Today the market has been expanded to include adults.

CONFLICTS OF INTEREST

Advertisements in medical journals support the infrastructure of clinical trial results published in peer review journals. Articles may be ghostwritten by account executives in public relations agencies, according to a leading medical journal editor. When the American Medical Association got wind of this ten years ago, they conducted a survey of the journals and found that 11 percent of the articles had been ghostwritten and ruled that it should not occur. The PR firms where the ghostwriters work do not invent science: they take the information from clinical trials funded by Pharma and position it in mass media using a physician's byline. Many aspects of this scenario seem unbelievable, yet it happens. Wyeth hired ghostwriters to promote the lethal diet drug fen-phen, according to litigation documents. Similar evidence was submitted in legal trials against Neurotonin, an epilepsy drug manufactured by Warner-Lambert.[75]

In a demonstration of a more subtle, yet legal manipulation of persuasive evidence, Angell alleged that in publishing scientific results in peer-review medical journals, it may be possible that editors select articles compatible with companies advertising in the journal, because ad revenues are "the life-support for research journal publishing."[76] This is a powerful statement from a respected and distinguished physician who worked for twenty years as editor of a peer-review journal relied on as authoritative by journalists. Though the annual expenditure on advertising in medical journals by drug companies is small compared to other areas, the potential for its influence on doctors is not as significant as its potential for influence in the mass media, which picks up without question the information published there as scientific, objective, and unbiased belies their potential for influence on physicians. Ethics rules in peer-review medical journals have mandated disclosure of the conflict of interest by physicians, and disclosure of all funding sources is now required in a headnote. Despite recent advances in this regard, the problem persists, especially in conditions involving branded neurological symptoms about which little is known, where medication is widespread and scientific data is still contested.

For example, in September 2006, the editor of the *Journal of Neuropsychopharmacology*, Charles Nemeroff, an Emory University psychiatry department chair, stepped down from his role as editor after he wrote a favorable review of a new device for treating depression but did not disclose his financial ties to the manufacturer of the device. The device, implanted in the chest, "delivered mild electrical impulses to the vagus nerve in the neck," according to David Armstrong, the *Wall Street Journal* reporter who covered the story. The article in the medical journal declared the device "a promising and well-tolerated intervention that is effective in a subset of patients with treatment-resistant depression," according to Armstrong. In addition to Nemeroff, seven of the other eight authors of the article were academics who served as consultants to the maker of the device, and one was an employee of the manufacturer, Cyberonics, Inc., of Houston.[77]

In another recent example, a doctor presented research results to a conference of cardiologists, showing the benefits of a blood filtering device rather than diuretics to remove excess fluid from patients with heart failure. The doctor did disclose to the audience that she was a paid consultant with stock in the company that made the device, but did not reveal that the manufacturer had made contributions ($180,000) to the nonprofit research foundation that had overseen the study. The nonprofit foundation was an arm of the for-profit medical group that employed the doctor in a group practice of more than fifty physicians. *The New York Times* saw this evidence as part of a trend, something now attracting regulators' attention, rather than a singular instance of confused ethics: "Around the country, doctors in private practice have set up tax-exempt charities into which drug companies and medical device makters are, with little fanfare, pouring donations . . . add[ing] up to a million dollars a year."[78] The *Times* noted that critics have seized on this as a form of "relationship funding," where industry promotes its wares indirectly, cultivating doctors by contributing to charities that in turn oversee clinical research whose results are disseminated through talks to medical conferences, in continuing doctor education programs paid for by the industry, and in publications in peer-review journals.

Some physicians think that conflict of interest is a good thing, as one doctor was quoted in *The New York Times* as saying—that the types of experts who are really influential usually do have conflicts of interest, which shows they are listened to by a broad number of publics. When one physician published an article in the trade press, *Physician's Weekly*, about "aspirin resistance," the subject had been well trod by numerous research articles in medical journals. Another physician connected the emergence of the disease "aspirin resistance" with the introduction of the drug Plavix. He projected that the potential market for aspirin substitutes might involve 30 percent of Americans, or about 25 million people who take aspirin for heart attack prevention. Aspirin resistance describes a possible condition among some people who do not benefit from the 81 mg a day of aspirin prescribed to reduce the likelihood of heart attacks, and who would need other anticlotting medication. "Fears of aspirin resistance have boosted sales of the anticlotting pill Plavix, the world's second best-selling drug after cholesterol drug Lipitor." Medicare reported twice the tests to measure aspirin resistance between 2002 and 2004, when there were forty-three thousand lab tests conducted. As Armstrong of the *Wall Street Journal* reported, Dr. Simon's research is supported by Accumetrics, Inc., a company that makes tests to measure aspirin resistance, and he is also a paid consultant and speaker for Schering Plough, manufacturer of a drug being tested as an antidote for aspirin resistance, which also supports his research. "Expertise" and "medical authority" have become synonymous with "influence."

When the editor of the trade weekly was questioned by the reporter, he acknowledged that a trade publication "does not disclose conflicts of interest, even when they know about them," as they did in the case of the article on aspirin resistance. On the contrary, the editor commented, they used the information in order to solicit advertising for the publication from the drug companies near or alongside the article. A convergence of social and economic forces makes a cultural climate possible where trade and peer review, for-profit and nonprofit, advertising and education are increasingly blurred.

Of course, most physicians are not so blind to the problem of public trust. Armstrong reported that Dr. Eric Topol, considered a leading expert, was quoted in an Accumetrics press release, saying that the test for aspirin resistance was a prototype for the "future of individualized medicine," though Dr. Topol is reported as not having given either the quote or the permission to use the quote. At the time he was a paid consultant to Accumetrics and two other firms, plus a paid consultant to Bristol-Myers, Sanofi-Aventis, and Lilly, all developing aspirin-resistance medications. Undoubtedly, the quote was crafted by a wordsmith account executive responsible for the drafting the release. Now Dr. Topol has cut all ties with industry to avoid the appearance of conflict, according to Armstrong. Authors of a "special report" in the American Heart Association journal *Circulation* in 2004, warning that aspirin resistance research was "unsubstantiated," had ties to Bayer, but the omission of this conflict of interest was blamed on "production error" by the editor, as Armstrong reported.[79]

Old-fashioned advertising is only one means of influence in the Medicated Public Square. In addition, old-school lobbying tactics such as "expensive dinners for physicians where research studies . . . are discussed" still flourish. In the case of Lexapro, manufactured by Forest Laboratories, Melody Peterson of *The New York Times* reported that "[j]ust days after the FDA approved Lexapro, twenty doctors were invited to dine at one of Manhattan's most expensive restaurants, and they were paid $500 each to feast on tournados of beef and cabernet sauvignon." The FDA issued warnings to drug companies in recently proposed guidelines that cash or gifts to doctors to persuade their prescribing medications would become illegal.[80] Medical education for physicians is another point where potential conflict of interest and persuasive tactics come under fire. The Pharma industry paid for an estimated 57 to 90 percent of the costs of doctors attending the 686 accredited continuing medical education programs, an estimated market of $700 to $900 million a year.[81]

Celebrity name dropping of a branded condition also can cultivate "intimacy." Celebrity endorsements of a drug occur in news interviews rather than in testimonials attached to an advertisement, a more subtle PR mechanism for delivering the message. Traditionally, celebrities have been used as spokespersons representing a particular brand. But they have become "central figures" paid between $20,000 and $2 million in campaigns to change public perception about normalcy. Recently, after Jane Pauley announced she had "bipolar disorder" in a book about her life, *The New York Times* sought her testimony for an advertising supplement to the paper for Eli Lilly and other manufacturers of psychotherapeutic drugs, in an interview that resulted in her suing the newspaper for deception.[82] Young sports figures have replaced the aging Bob Dole to market "erectile dysfunction," and the once supermodel Lauren Hutton, used to position a "loss" of estrogen as endemic to normal female aging, has been replaced by a homelier figure, the former flying nun, Sally Fields, in kitchen table talk about medicine in a "self-care" regimen where a monthly rather than weekly dose of Fosamax rebuilds bone. Maybe the advertisement caught the attention of Hollywood television producers of the medical soap opera *ER*: Fields appeared in that popular drama at the same time her advertisements were running.

CUSTOMIZING DOCTOR APPEALS

Marketing to doctors requires a different set of tactics than those used to reach consumers. Rather than create pseudo-intimacy, marketers want to "drill down," customizing their approach to suit information about individual doctors. Using data from hospitals and the American Medical Association, strategies for customer retention have developed based on the "strategic value of each physician," an attitude cluster based on their degree of "aggressiveness" about prescribing drugs.[83]

The same privacy guarantees extended to patients through the Health Insurance Portability and Accountability Act (HIPAA) are not available to doctors. The Drug Enforcement Administration has registration numbers, and state medical license numbers; pharmacies have internal identifiers, all of which could be cross-listed with other databases about physician identity in a software program such as the one sold under the Physician Profiler trademark. Based on this data, sales reps and medical liaisons could target the nonprescribing physicians with incentives and "disease awareness kits," and "patient education programs" developed by leading health care public relations experts at Grey, Edelmann, or the half dozen other global communication firms.[84] This technology merges micromarketing, advertising, sales techniques, and software. From a strategic standpoint, such information has powerful reach and proactive trend-setting advantages.

In a midsummer, 2006 "Perspective" piece in the *New England Journal of Medicine*, Robert Steinbrook, M.D., outlined the process where information mined from pharmacies is matched with American Medical Association data, compiled by data bank companies and sold to pharmaceutical manufacturers.[85] The AMA's Physician Masterfile of licensed doctors contains 820,000 names, including current and historical data on physicians from the time of their undergraduate medical education; the database includes AMA members, nonmembers, and graduates of foreign medical schools living in the United States. In 2005 the sale of this information brought $44.5 million to the AMA, about 16 percent of its total revenue. The AMA requires that Pharma companies using this data must "police" their sales force. The California Medical Association is testing a program where doctors can compare their own data with an industry profile of the most heavily prescribed medication categories. Gallup polled the membership for AMA in 2004, and reported that nearly a quarter of doctors were unaware of this practice by the AMA; 66 percent opposed the release of the data to sales representatives, and 77 percent said they wanted the option to block the information being made available to sales representatives. A drug needs to become a "best seller" in the first nine months, because patents are "on the clock," especially if the FDA review has been lengthy. To reach that goal, consumers must be readied by prelaunch publicity to "ask their doctor," and the physician must be prepared as well to prescribe when consumers request the drug.[86]

Critics of the scandalous conflicts of interest among doctors and aggressive target marketing of physicians point to the "lowering of baseline standards" for such conditions as high blood pressure, blood glucose, osteoporosis, cholesterol, and obesity as the place where self-interests and corporate interests coincide to expand the potential market by normalizing the inevitability of predisease states.[87] Yet advocates for pharmaceutical marketing argue that this trend is a violation of ethical standards and, further, may serve a broader public health purpose. Some people may actually alter their lifestyle, exercise more, and eat better foods because of the information disseminated through the mass media. There is also a logic for the prescription culture as the nation ages, and a rationality to the conclusion among some critics that certain prescriptions will be considered as universal as vitamins. Those drugs may include vasodilators, blood thinners, antidepressants, and sleep medicine. But this is a market forecast based on the continued strength of the trend in selling the idea of sickness to a well population. Not everyone is buying in. A sizable, growing, and statistically significant cohort of resistors are turning to complementary medicine and rational drug therapy.

SOCIAL COSTS

The complementary and alternative medicine movement is estimated to exceed $60 billion a year—a mere David with a slingshot before the Goliath of Big Pharma. For contrast, drug companies had combined global sales of $217 billion, and that is just the companies based in the United States.[88] Of that amount, about $34 billion was spent on marketing globally, exporting American brand values and identity along with the push across cultural borders. Angell alleged that of the companies belonging to the trade association for pharmaceutical manufacturers, slightly more than 35 percent of all employees were in the marketing function, amounting to a line item of about $54 billion.[89] That would be nearly the annual budget for all of CAM. Angell estimated that marketing was twice the cost of research and development, and that disproportionate expenditure on marketing tripled since 1997, when Congress and the Food and Drug Administration made changes in direct-to-consumer advertisements in all forms of mass media, resulting in a forty percent increase in television advertising alone. Mintzes forecast that the direct-to-consumer advertising of pharmaceuticals would reach nearly $345 million by 2008.[90] Congress required that all advertisements be cleared for fairness by the FDA, but the publicity market is outpacing the bureaucracy, so some ads have been run, only to be later sanctioned. The pharmaceutical industry needs faster clearance to accommodate media buying and campaign planning. After the withdrawal of several medications because of lethal side effects and insufficient warnings about side effects, and no doubt because of the slow pace of FDA approval of advertisements, pharmaceutical companies increased their overall spending on advertising by nearly 10 percent, reaching $2.46 billion in the most recent six-month period before this book's publication, but they allocated it across mass media differently. After the industry adopted voluntary guidelines to improve the accuracy and balance of ads, and to disclose fully the side effects of drugs, TNS Media Intelligence reported that television ads were down slightly, in favor of magazine advertising; newspaper ads still remained a small percentage of their overall ad budget.

Research on the FDA revealed that in the review process the majority of letters sent to manufacturers cited "disease mongering" in the misrepresentation of disease or an exaggeration of the treatment, and off-label promotion broadly interpreting symptoms.[91] Household brand names were cited for violations of fairness, including those that later became targets of lawsuits for unsafe drugs, including Celebrex, Vioxx, Enbrel, Levitra, Paxil, Strattera, and Viagra. According to the FDA, these advertisements "omitted risks," or made a pitch for "unsubstantiated effectiveness and superiority claims," or "overstated effectiveness" and "minimized risks."[92] For the first time in thirty years, the FDA made changes in drug labeling, which an editorial in the New England Journal of Medicine called a "regulatory time bomb," a clause that would further "shield drug makers from legal action," and one added after the close of the five-year public comment period.[93] William Shrank, M.D., of Harvard Medical School, stressed that the FDA missed the most vital point: the delivery of risk and benefit information to doctors.[94]

As this book is being written, the front-page Wall Street news about the pharmaceutical industry is what the press perceives as closed-door negotiations with the FDA, about increasing the industry's "user fee," the tariff paid to those who review the advertisements. The pharmaceutical industry wanted the FDA to speed the approval process of advertisements, to twelve months at most. The industry pays fees to the FDA when the companies file for the initial patent and approval application, scaled according to the size of the company and the number of drugs currently under review. After nearly a century of nonindustry, taxpayer support, David Kessler, M.D., then FDA commissioner, introduced the idea of the Pharma industry financially contributing to the FDA, the regulator mandated with its oversight. In the past decade, industry support for the agency grew from 7 percent to 53 percent of its total annual budget, or dollars, from $9 million to $232 million. The industry is negotiating with the FDA to increase that amount to cover 65 percent of its annual budget, or an additional $100 million. These are costs that manufacturers must recover from consumers in the price of drugs. Every five years the industry and agency renegotiate the user fees, and according to journalist Mathews, the highly "secretive" policy process subject to congressional approval is under increasing scrutiny by elected officials. The FDA wants the industry to pay for its surveillance of imported, counterfeit drugs, while the industry would like the number of staff reviewing advertisements increased from thirty-four to fifty, though that view is not unanimous, and more advance notice than thirty days is to be required for modification of labels before a new drug is launched.[95] Mintzes argued that government protections are "piecemeal" and "largely ineffective."[96]

Currently, all these details about how industry interacts with government have a profound effect on the cost of drugs as well as broader issues in American health policy. Lobbyists have a significant role in shaping these matters that usually escape the attention of the American consumer. Many are "revolving door" lobbyists, who have built expertise in the finer points of law by being lawmakers: once elected officials, they move from the congressional to the regulatory side. In the current negotiations about user fees, for example, "several" of the industry representatives are "former FDA" officials, "sitting across the table from current government officials at the agency's offices in suburban Washington in meetings that have been going on for months," according to news reports.[97] Both current and past commissioners assert that there has been neither "compromise" nor a "lowering of the regulatory bar," and they observed that "consumer groups" and the general public both have the right to comment on an arrangement that the *Wall Street Journal* calls "complex." Yet there is no oversight about the degree to which the pharmaceutical industry has supported the "consumer groups" who offer comment. Neither the Securities and Exchange Commission nor the Federal Communications Commission negotiate user fees directly with the industries they regulate.

The FDA review of drug promotion is at the heart of the Medicated Public Square because its power to shape the culture and influence popular receptivity to the product escapes most consumers and journalists. Watchdogs tracking the industry have taken notice. A 2003 report by Ralph Nader's group Public Citizen charged that the pharmaceutical industry employed 700 lobbyists when bills were in Congress that would have the net effect of lowering the price of drugs. In that effort, of the 675 lobbyists in 138 firms, 26 were former members of Congress and another 342 had "revolving door" connections between their government employment and lobbying. The *Report on Drug Lobbying* also found that the industry spent $91.4 million on lobbying in addition to $50 million in advertising and public relations, direct mail, telemarketing, advocacy groups, and academic research, up 12 percent from the previous year. Since 1997, the industry spent $478 million on lobbying the federal government, $30 million on political advertising in the last election cycle, $48.6 million donated to the election campaigns of key elected representatives, and $3.4 million to political action committees.

In the 2003 push to privatize the Medicare drug benefit, PhRMA spent $77 million at the federal level and $48 million at the state level to change the law. An additional $12 million subsidized health groups that supported PhRMA's stance on the drug issue, and $9.4 million was spent on advertising and public relations, with another $1 million to "'create an intellectual echo chamber' of economists and 'thought leaders' who oppose any federal regulation of drug prices"; $550,000 more was set aside for "placement of op-eds and articles by third parties." The net effect, according to the Nader group report, was to hold back cost reform and to permit corporations to extend their patent protection for new drugs.[98]

AGING MINDS AND THE NEXT FRONTIER

Reading into PhRMA's strategic materials, it looks as if the drug industry is banking on a sizable cohort of Americans losing their minds as they age, and some have suggested that cognitive impairment and dementia will be the next market to be expanded. It is hard not to gasp when read-ing these materials, or to hear Woody Allen's famous one-liner, that he did not mind dying, so long as he didn't have to be there. Currently, 241 new medicines are in development for psychiatric and neurologic diseases, which are estimated to "cost Americans $100 billion annually in lost pro-ductivity, medical expenses, sick leave, property and environmental dam-age."[99] According to PhRMA CEO Billy Tauzin, 42 are in development to treat Alzheimer's disease, "which afflicts 4.5 million Americans" or 1 in 10 people over 65, and "nearly half of those over 85." A close reading of PhMRA's list shows a broad range of "indicators" from dementia to mild cognitive impairment; most of the drugs are in the Phase I or II sta-tus. Italian scientists Maggini, Vanacore, and Raschetti argued recently that "cholinesterase inhibitors" are another instance of drugs looking for a disease, and that bragging rights about cures for dementia using these types of drugs were based on faulty clinical trials: "Drug companies have invested heavily in developing treatments for Alzheimer's . . . then were actively involved in expanding the market to other forms." The most developed is Aricept, produced by Pfizer, which is widely advertised, though industry records indicate that the "application has been submit-ted." In addition, the industry is developing 21 medicines for Parkinson's disease, "which affects 1.5 million"; medicines for brain tumors, based on the industry estimate of 359,000 people with primary brain tumors; 13 medicines for stroke; 11 for migraines, which they estimate affect 28 million people or 13 percent of the population; 27 medicines for multiple sclerosis, which afflicts 400,000; and 13 medicines for epilepsy, based on industry estimates of 2 million with that disease. Simple relief from pain is the largest area of medicine for neurologic disorders; 62 medicines are being developed, based on an estimated 57 percent of adults with chronic pain. The trend is toward compound medications: from once a day to once a week to monthly, or to combine effects, such as both pain and sleep. This will require fewer pills, with higher dosages, resulting in greater cost efficiency for the industry, although the advertisements tout that the compound medications are designed with the consumer in mind.

All these estimates for the future market for these diseases listed by PhRMA are "presented in cooperation with" twenty-six associations dedicated to specific diseases, from the American Headache Society to the Michael J. Fox Foundation for Parkinson's Research, the Tourette Syndrome Association, and the National Chronic Pain Outreach Association, though PhRMA prints a disclaimer at the end of their report that the cooperative arrangement does not imply the disease or patient association's endorsement of the industry.[100]

Moynihan's argument, distilled from Payer and Parry, is that promoting disease exacerbates anxiety and influences how people think about life. Wolinsky called the United States the "epicenter" for drug and drug-marketing innovation. Payer, Parry, Moynihan, and Wolinsky observed that routine human conditions increasingly are being defined as disease. Along with the invention of new diseases, the marketing paradigm of medical consumption has been patterned after other consumer products, without questioning the profound spiritual differences between things people do not require, and medicine, which they do require. As consumption is redefined, and with it the collective ideas about health, so, too, are medical authority, spiritual advice, and other cultural attributes of American identity. Applbaum declared that the contemporary drug-marketing environment is a "direct continuation of the nineteenth-century patent medicine advertising" condemned by William James. Applbaum attributed the growth of the pharmaceutical culture to beliefs about the free market, based on the insatiability and limitlessness of human needs and wants, and the popular belief put into choice making about things, about purchasing as the satisfaction that will ameliorate suffering. Along with these deeply rooted cultural beliefs is a hope in the free market, as a source of American ingenuity and innovation, and in health, as things that will ultimately serve the common good. "Transforming the identity of patients into consumers empowers them with the ideals of the free market and of choices that reflect their individuality and ability to make cost-effective decisions," Applbaum argued, but this "conversion from patient to consumer also paves the way for the erosion of the doctor's role as expert."[101] Medicine, Media, and Religion converge as climates of belief shaped by personal and cultural reality. If people cannot trust doctors and the pharmaceutical industry that creates the medicines they prescribe, they will seek refuge in alternatives. These may be in other styles of healing, or in a type of spiritual authority that also gives medical perspectives about religion.

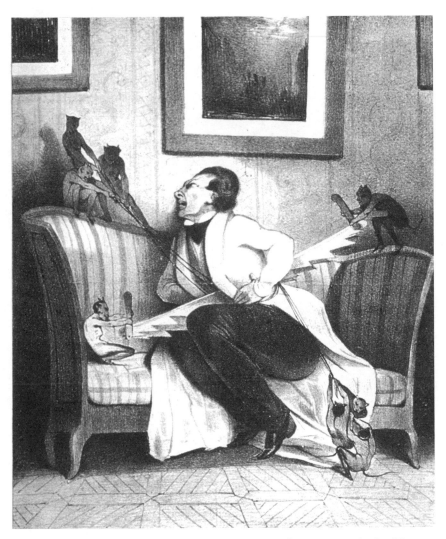

Figure 5.3: L'imagination (Imagination of a Disease), by Honoré
Daumier. Original caption reads: "La Colique. Hola! hola!. . . hola!
le ventre!. . . hola!" Published in Le Charivari (Paris, ca. 1800s), 6.
Courtesy of the National Library of Medicine.

CONCLUSION

Ideas embedded in the American philosophical and metaphysical culture historically have positioned the field of professional medicine as an enemy of faith, alleging that science was incompatible with the intuitive intelligence of the believer. Although twentieth-century physicians strove to differentiate themselves from the spiritual messages of ministers, a significant number of respected doctors and religious leaders in the new millennium are seeking to understand ways in which medicine and spirituality converge. In complementary and alternative medicine, particularly in mind-body approaches to healing and to health, ideas about the introspective power of the mind to influence the biochemistry of the body are experiencing a resurgence. Mass media, which is responsible for popularizing ideas in surface culture, has featured historical concepts as new, while advertising that supports the economic infrastructure of the news industry offers a branded awareness of pharmaceuticals. All of these elements converge as parts of the integrated social economy of medicine.

The two strains in American culture about science and religion were framed by William James, in the chapter on the "Religion of Healthy Mindedness," in *Varieties of Religious Experience*, where he claimed in lectures circa 1901–1902 that there were two kinds of people in America, the once-born and twice-born.[1] His theory about two kinds of people pertains to how we think collectively as a nation today about health as well as religion. It is fair to reiterate James and say that there are two kinds of people in America: those who think ideas about the role of religion in medicine are fundamental, ancient, and historical, and those who think these ideas, constructed through mass media, are born again. And there are two camps in American commercial culture: the science of molecular and biological discovery, and the science of public opinion engineering.

The challenge of complementary and alternative approaches to traditional medical arts lies in their proposition that scientific rationalism is not incompatible with spirituality. Attitudes comparable to those expressed in mind-body medicine can be found in the literature of Christian mysticism, transcendental idealism, Buddhism, and in early writing about modern psychology, which coalesced in the Mind-Cure movements at the turn of the twentieth century. While "not everyone can pray," as James observed, it would be fair to say that everyone can imagine, and in a culture where anxiety is a pandemic, that means everyone has an equal opportunity to fret. The imagination of disease and the anxiety and worry that cause disease is at the heart of the persuasive public opinion science of advertising illness in order to sell pharmaceuticals as a universal cure. Prescribing faith practices based on mental discipline, contemplative science, and prayer are antithetical to the imagination of disease.

Advertising pills and public education campaigns about disease are not merely about pharmaceutical products; they are about creating the perception that the product is "required," and as a consequence they have an impact on culture. So the product is more than just the chemical components of the drug. Its branding is connected with the culture of consumerism and the larger worldview about mortality, and so it is fair to say that such advertisements have spiritual content, in the sense that they express an anxiety about death and advocate a set of moral values that have to do with where the audience places its trust: in spiritual ideas about the healing of the body, or in the messages of advertising. In the sense that pharmaceutical advertising is connected with public perceptions about and confidence in medical authority, widespread public distrust of the drug industry because of negative publicity extends to its perception of the medical profession. In a converged economy where electronic news, Internet information, advertising, and public relations are all tying together the role of rational choice by consumers to the hope of wellness, the result is a vernacular of pseudoscience, a cultural vocabulary of brand names associated with promises and longevity, of youth, promises that transcend psychodemographic divisions of the population according to ethnicity or denomination.

Williams James observed in his early twentieth-century lectures that "the creed" of positive thinkers connected traditional dualistic distinctions drawn from Christianity about the higher and the lower self, egotism, and doubt as a philosophical current that had the potential to affirm the complacency of the overly certain about the life of the spirit and, in doing so, undermined real science and real religion. Surface culture is made up of the ideas that spin rapidly across popular awareness through mass media, while deeper cultural beliefs shift more slowly and sometimes at a glacial pace. So while it may seem to the news industry that great innovations are occurring, if we look more deeply and deconstruct the images, certain values and attitudes remained unchanged. Fear replaced self-centeredness in defining sin, in James's interpretation of the religion of healthy-mindedness. He denounced the proselytizing of mind-cure writers who engendered the "misery-habit" and "martyr-habit" as part of the "worry" about disease conjured up by physicians. Today, the pharmaceutical industry has taken over that role, cultivating worry about the possibility of disease while offering its products as a cure. The revenue stream from disease advertising supports the journalism industry, which also uses fear appeals in reporting, accentuating the existing anxiety about threats, by breaking stories about pseudo-science distilled from press releases.

The power of faith and the power of the imagination have played and continue to operate as a cultural agent in society. Faith dictates how we heal; the imagination determines how we consume. More than a century ago, Mary Baker Eddy used publishing in a way envied by her critics, even those adepts in the modern media such as Mark Twain and Joseph Pulitzer. In publishing her religious books and newspapers, she employed what would become the "Method of the Future." In modernism, that became the belief invested in the product that created its value. As Besant wrote, the "performance" of the book as a product occurred not in the writing, advertising, or selling in bookstores; it occurred when the public bought into its world and used the words and the imaginative scope contained in the book as their own. There was a psychological process of adoption that contributed to adaptation, to buying into the values implicit in the product. That is selling via branding, to get the consumer to think of himself or herself as a participant in the larger cultural story by transference of the image in the press to their own identity and, then, by extension to identify with the disease or predisease state, given rationality through repetition of the language in commercial speech. This transference of identity is lived out in consumer rituals, in the choices purchasers make at the drugstore. The same "method" shapes the advertising of disease today. When Mark Twain sat in his library at his home, with Besant's book on his lap and a pencil in his hand, ruminating on his profits from *Adventures of Huckleberry Finn* and comparing his royalties and production costs with Mary Baker Eddy's, he predicted that the method of the future would put authors, ministers, doctors, and readers in the same economic boat. Unless buyers thought a product was "required," it wouldn't sell, whether it was media, religion, or medicine.

James criticized Eddy because she had flatly declared "a lie" the imagination of disease in her book *Science and Health*. Yet she was in good company, because in his view, the other culprits who contributed to the popularity at the turn of the twentieth century of current ideas about religion and health were the writers of the four Gospels, with the many miracle cures of Jesus, the New England Transcendentalism of Emerson, and what James called "spiritism" with its "messages of law and progress and development," as well as Hinduism.

In the nineteenth century, he thought, it was not only the primitive state of medicine but also the religious doctrines that contributed to the nation's anxiety. James's description of "mind-cure religion" treated it as reactionary, a swing of the pendulum against the popularization of worries about being a sinner, a "religion of chronic anxiety . . . in the evangelical churches of England and America." The religion of healthy-mindedness encompassed, he wrote, "an intuitive belief . . . in the conquering efficacy of courage, hope, and trust, and a correlative contempt for doubt, fear, worry, and all nervously precautionary states of mind." The rapid expansion of this positivism in religion and medicine, or, more aptly, the role of faith and fear in a psychology of belief, is the philosophical thread linking contemporary schools of alternative medicine, and mind-body prescriptions for faith with the ideas about the power of mind during the era of James.

James captured the essence of the American spiritualities, which expressed a "practical" character trait. Extending his observation to the present, one might say that there is not only a therapeutic culture within which the contemporary perspectives about religion and medicine thrive, mixing self-interest with self-reliance in an understanding of both science and medicine, but also a utilitarian strain, a pragmatics involved. Undoubtedly, people turn to religion for its therapeutic value if it is prescribed, so within that context, belief itself becomes a product. James wrote, "The deliberate adoption of a healthy-minded attitude has proven possible to many who never supposed they had it in them. . . . One hears of the 'Gospel of Relaxation,' of the 'Don't Worry Movement,' of people who repeat to themselves, 'Youth, health, vigor!' when dressing in the morning, as their motto for the day. Complaints about the weather are getting to be forbidden in many households." He argued that religious and medical authorities were slow to recognize the power and persuasive efficacy of this type of positivist thinking. James predicted that the ability of those who were in this camp to write well and to explain their ideas about positive, purpose-driven spiritual outlooks that were efficacious without getting into anything sticky like grace were "evidently bound to develop still farther, both speculatively and practically." As the high tide of medical and spiritual advice books on the best-seller lists today demonstrates, James was right on the money. Though there will always be skeptics, he allowed, the popularity of the converged religions of healthy-mindedness in American culture constituted "so large a group" at the time, James thought, that they "form a psychic type to be studied with respect." The purpose of this book is to assert that they still do.

Beneath the controversies—the headlines about drug recalls and litigation against manufacturers for violations of drug safety, the streaming visual communication that fuels the imagination of disease unless checked by resistance—are questions fundamental to American culture. Above all, Americans in a democratic order believe in freedoms—of expression, of religion, of the right to happiness. After all, Americans in a religiously pluralistic nation believe in certain universals, their rights to health and longevity and to the health care infrastructure that includes hospitals and safe pharmaceuticals. Choices people make about their own health as consumers of medical information, transmitted and based on science translated by the news media, and choices people make about whether or not medical or scientific authority trumps that of religious authority, are taken on balance with their political and economic beliefs.

The architecture of this book has proceeded by juxtaposition of past and present, to elucidate how the current debates about medicine, media, and faith evolved, and how universal truths about our human need to prefer happiness and avoid suffering have entered middle-brow culture through mass media—a mediated vernacular that has been adopted and used as a commodity. The enlightenment provided by history is that we can see our earlier reflections and understand better the family resemblances that demonstrate, no matter how far we have come, that there is still the genome to consider. Is it rational, investigative, clinical science that shapes our belief about the role of the mind in health, or what defines the physical limits of the spiritual intelligence? Is our collective unconscious rattled by anxiety about health that creates climates of pseudo-beliefs that shape our science? Do media workers have the education necessary to interpret scientific facts for the public, rather than simply transmit press releases from publicity agents representing the financial interests of research scientists and pharmaceutical manufacturers? What psychological factors trigger belief in electronic images and messages among the unchurched? Traditionally, we tend to think not only about science and religion as separate realms, but also about mass media as bereft of the influence or content to shape beliefs that penetrate the deeper culture having to do with ideas about mortality and the spirit. But the central argument of this book is that these segments of culture are integrally related, and interdependent, shaping one another as well as the progressive and reactionary notions that define the climates of opinion and rational choices in each.

Given the number of current legal challenges to the drug industry, one questions the pace at which clinical trials are conducted and government approval is granted. Perhaps more clinical trial evidence should be required, or the FDA approval process should be more deliberative, less open to the influence of lobbying and advertising. Perhaps the staff should be increased, providing more oversight. Perhaps the off-label uses of drugs for serious illness applied to ailments formerly treated by over-the-counter drugs should be less secretive and made more visible for public consideration by thought leaders in the scientific and medical community. Perhaps as a profession doctors should distance themselves from the pharmaceutical manufacturers' image and from any implication of a conflict of interest, whether that be in funding research or in collecting fees. But the resolution of these controversies is a debate that seldom makes its way into the "Naked" or "Medicated" Public Square.

Problems about "medicalizing" women persist, nearly always raising the larger moral questions for our age, just as they did in the age of Sophia Peabody and Mary Baker Eddy in experimental cures for the pains of childbirth and toxic cures for hysteria. For example, consider the cultural implications of a vaccine against cervical cancer, now approved for girls as young as nine years old in the United States and exported globally to third-world countries; the cure is considered to be a "universal" vaccine against sexually transmitted diseases. News stories about this vaccine's introduction showed mothers consenting for their preteen daughters, saying that this is a tremendous medical advance. News coverage about the introduction of the vaccine did not question the side effects of the drug, either physically or morally. Nor did they raise the factor of cultural conditioning that sanctioned a medical product as "required," part of the cultural story that normalizes sexual relations as "natural" for school-age children who do not have the intellectual capacity to solve problems, understand history or literature, or in many cases have the basic reading and math skills necessary to hold a job and contribute to the economy when they mature.[2] Consider another "required" product, the "French pill RU486," the notorious "morning after" pill that was both ingested and inserted and proved life-threatening, now replaced by an over-the-counter "Plan B" medication that is the equivalent of one month's birth control pills in one pill, routinely reported in the press without any discussion of the long-term health impact of such powerful doses of hormones. Nowhere in the Medicated Public Square have questions been raised about the side effects, not just physically but also morally, of long-term use of these drugs on the spiritual or public culture. The process of normalizing the behavioral fringe expands the domain of the therapeutic culture, while the mainstream that may object to its prescriptions on religious grounds is distracted by other partisan issues about health debated in the mass media.

More congressional oversight of drug safety and a more "rational drug therapy," to borrow the European phrase, is called for. This might tip the balance between the global power of advertising that normalizes fear through required product placement, and the lack of science training among journalists that makes them complicit in such a media economy by disseminating press releases verbatim or without critical questioning and investigation. Because lawsuits make good headlines, though they undermine public trust in the pharmaceutical industry, Americans are unsure what to believe about medicine and waver between the emotional pull of media and the harsh realities of American public policy about health care.

U.S. policies about direct-to-consumer (DTC) drug advertising should be consistent with global practices. Though even the advertising trade press admits the practice of direct-to-consumer advertising is controversial, the United States persists in being the Lone Ranger, along with the small population of New Zealand, in sanctioning as legal the direct-to-consumer marketing of drugs on television. The claim of "public education about health" is more about branding than it is about informing, and that DTC advertising should be treated like tobacco and alcohol advertising, or banned altogether; but putting that genie back in the bottle is unrealistic given the "required" revenue stream it provides the struggling journalism industry, and the competitive impetus for drug innovation by the lucrative pharmaceutical industry. So where is the Golden Mean, the Middle Way, between the drive for profits and consumer protection in this ethical dilemma where real harm can come to the consumer through DTC advertising—if not through the products themselves, then by universalizing predisease conditions, and contributing to the anxiety or "precautionary" beliefs of Americans? The bottom line is that climates of belief about intangibles are constructed through the selling of commodities, a process that has pervaded every aspect of high culture, of medicine and religion as well as middlebrow and low culture, and that branded awareness of things, from athletic shoe logos to anti-stroke medication, is made possible through global mass media enterprise in converged electronic news, advertising, and public relations industries.

A public health policy that is the result of revolving-door special interests, where members of the U.S. government move into industry, capitalizing on their track record as elected officials and profiting from prior connections with political decision makers, is a sleeper issue, one seldom talked about by campaigning politicians or by the journalists who cover the electoral or health beat; it remains the "secret" of the Medicated Public Square. The close-knit relationship between the FDA and the drug industry it is meant to govern should be extricated, and laws should prohibit a revolving-door relationship between elected officials engaged in rule making to protect consumers and their ability to go to work for the drug industry, profiting from having been a political "authority."[3]

Increasing numbers of people reject the traditional medical industry in favor of complementary and alternative approaches, and an increasing number of medical doctors accept the idea about the role of prayer in healing and in preventing disease. In a climate of distrust for Big Pharma, advertising drugs deepens the public doubt about the pharmaceutical industry, its concerns for the safety of its products versus its drive for profits, and by extension, the doctors who do the prescribing of these drugs. Mass media campaigns are responsible for changing attitudes about how people think about their own health, and the meaning of a healing presence.

Further, if a recent *US News & World Report* magazine cover feature is to be considered indicative of a trend, the news media has become interested in more than the shift to mind-body medicine; their interest is piqued by brain research and neuroscience delving into the metaphysical. As the introduction of this book discussed, in 2003, *Newsweek* celebrated Dr. Harold Koenig's work in exploring religion and health. Three years later almost to the day, the October 23, 2006 magazine cover of their competitor, US News & World Report, for a feature article about how new research "is challenging our most cherished ideas of self and human spirit."[4] The running headline blazed over the image of a woman's face. Not unlike the 2003 Newsweek cover that was about Dr. Harold Koenig but featured a generic patient, the everywoman about to entrust her life to the hospital, the same disembodied female face on the cover of US News & World Report floated in a starry cyberspace, in carefully applied lipstick. She is not looking up to heaven any longer, but straight out, level, eyeball to eyeball with the readers. Yet her eyes are as vacant as any cover model's or figure in an advertisement. The cover trumpets the news that scientists (all male) are discovering the identity of her soul and its boundaries, called the self. But the cover is not of the scientists; it is the of objectified woman whom scientists study. The prototype is again the white, middle-class, universal female medical consumer—who also is a public target for the ailing news magazine industry. The article is positioned as if to lift the readers' awareness about the current state of brain research, and the few pages devoted to the subject with photos describe the tip of the iceberg as centered in one California think tank, though brain research is going on worldwide. The revenue paying for the production costs of this glossy publication come from the center-fold of the magazine: in the October 2006 issue, for example, it would have been from a four-page advertisement for Ambien, the sleep disorder medication. The person depicted in the Ambien advertisement again looks familiar. Oddly enough, it is the same generic female face seen on the cover of the magazine. In the advertisement, she is less mythologized but equally bland, shown with a sleep mask, benefiting from the pharmaceutical product to induce the requisite good night's sleep, an increasingly rare commodity in a mediated culture of anxiety.

In our own day and age, how will resistance take shape to pharmaceutical culture and medicalizing consumers, particularly women, while leaving a third of the population without health insurance? In public policy debates in the Medicated Public Square? Will the business of advertising pseudoscience inspire some to join or to establish new religions in a formal resistance to medicine—religions that flourish precisely because they offer introspection and mental discipline as alternative sources of healing to the fatigue engendered by the anxiety of the mediated economy that relies on the imagination of disease and its concomitant fear? How will these influences and counterinfluences change the practice of American medicine for patients, how they think about the spiritual self, the boundaries of their souls as defined by scientists and reported by journalists? To what extent will media transform the role of faith in American medicine and in American religions? What role will knowledge of the ancient Eastern and Western religious traditions have on the contemporary practices of the healing arts? No matter which "side" prevails in this confluence of historical, social, philosophical, cultural, and economic forces—whether those who put hope into the constructed reality of the Medicated Public Square in which the imagination of disease plays a key role, or the ideas in mind-body medicine that prescribe ancient faith practices of contemplative science, albeit positioned in a therapeutic culture—the moral questions at the heart of the story remain to be answered, in the rational choices about faith made by the audience itself.

NOTES

Chapter 1

1 Claire Badaracco, "Pitfalls and Rewards of the Solo Editor: Sophia Peabody Hawthorne," *Resources in American Literary Studies* 11, no. 1 (1980): 91–100; and Badaracco, *The Cuba Journal, 1833–35, of Sophia Peabody Hawthorne*, from the holograph in the Berg Collection of the New York Public Library (UMI Press, Books on Demand; copies in the Library of Congress and the Berg Collection, 1982); Thomas Woody, *A History of Women's Education in the U.S.* (1929; repr. New York: Octagon, 1966); Elizabeth Palmer Peabody, "Female Education in Massachusetts," *Barnard's American Journal of Education* 30 (1880): 584; Elizabeth Palmer Peabody, *Record of a School: Exemplifying the General Principles of Spiritual Culture* (Boston: J. Monroe, 1835); A. Bronson Alcott, *Conversation with Children about the Gospels* (Boston: J. Monroe, 1836–37); Ann Douglas, *The Feminization of American Culture* (New York: Alfred Knopf, 1977).

2 Oliver Wendell Holmes, "Border Lines of Knowledge in Some Provinces of Medical Science: An Introductory Lecture, Delivered before the Medical Class of Harvard University, November 6, 1861" (Boston: Ticknor & Fields, 1862), 14.

3 Oliver Wendell Holmes, *Medical Essays, 1842–1882* (1883; repr. Boston: Houghton, Mifflin, 1891), 171, 211. See also Robley Dunglison, *The Medical Student; or, Aids to the Study of Medicine* (Philadelphia: Carey, Lea &

Blanchard, 1837), chap. 30. See also *American Medical Biography: Or Memoirs of Eminent Physicians who have Flourished in America to which is Affixed a Succinct History of Medical Science in the United States, from the First Settlement of the Country*, 2 vols. (Boston: Richardson & Lord and Cottons & Barnard, 1828).

4   Holmes, *Medical Essays*, 200. See also Oliver Wendell Holmes, *Puerperal Fever as a Private Pestilence* (Boston: Ticknor & Fields, 1835).

5   A. T. Schofield, *Nervousness: A Brief and Popular Review of the Moral Treatment of Disordered Nerves* (New York: Moffat, Yard & Co., 1909), 6–7.

6   Schofield, *Nervousness*, 8.

7   Schofield, *Nervousness*, 21.

8   R. Scott Stevenson, *Famous Illnesses in History* (London: Eyrie & Spottiswoode, 1962), 24–29.

9   Badaracco, *Cuba Journal*; Autographed Letter Signed (ALS) Walter Channing to Sophia A. Peabody, August 12, 1828; November 17, 1828; September 20, 1828; October 11, [1829?], Berg Collection; ALS Mary Peabody to Maria Chase, November 10, 1826; ALS Sophia Peabody to Maria Chase, January 9, 1828, Peabody Papers, Sophia Smith Collection. See also Megan Marshall, *The Peabody Sisters* (New York: Houghton Mifflin, 2005).

10   Schofield, *Nervousness*, 23.

11   Schofield, *Nervousness*, 32, 53, 69.

12   John S. Haller, *American Medicine in Transition, 1840–1910* (Urbana: University of Illinois Press, 1981), appendix B, 329.

13   Robert Fuller, *Alternative Medicine and American Religious Life* (New York: Oxford University Press, 1989), 14.

14   Fuller, *Alternative Medicine and American Religious Life*, 42. In 1810 Hahnemann published the work, *Organon of the Healing Art*, and in 1811, *Pure Materia Medica*. See Samuel Hahnemann, *Organon der rationellen Heilkunde* (Dresden: Arnoldischen Buchhandlung, 1810); Samuel Hahnemann, *Reine Arzneimittellehre* (Dresden: Arnoldischen Buchhandlung, 1811–1821).

15   Oliver Wendell Holmes, "Homeopathy and Its Kindred Delusions; Two Lectures Delivered before the Boston Society for the Diffusion of Useful Knowledge" (Boston: W. D. Ticknor, 1842), 1.

16   Holmes, "Homeopathy," 2.

17   Holmes, "Homeopathy," 39–40.

18   See also James Hamilton, Jr., *Observations on the Use and Abuse of Mercurial Medicines in Various Disease* (New York: Bliss & White, 1821), 255.

19   Hamilton, *Observations*, 276.

20 Amalie M. Kass, *Midwifery and Medicine in Boston: Walter Channing, M D, 1786–1876* (Boston: Northeastern University Press, 2002), 148–49. See also 321n24.

21 Kass, *Midwifery*, 150–51.

22 William Purrington, *A Review of Recent Legal Decisions Affecting Physicians, Dentists, Druggists and the Public Health, Together with a Brief for the Prosecution of Unlicensed Practitioners* (New York: E. B. Treat, 1899), 26.

23 Walter Channing, review of John Elwell, *A Medico-Legal Treatise on Malpractice and Medical Evidence, Comprising the Elements of Medical Jurisprudence, Boston Medical and Surgical Journal* 62, no. 12 (1860): 233–41.

24 Channing, review of Elwell, 234–35.

25 Walter Channing, *A Treatise on Etherization in Childbirth Illustrated by Five Hundred and Eighty-one Cases* (Boston: Ticknor & Fields, 1848), 6.

26 Channing, *Treatise*, 11, 2.

27 Channing, *Treatise*, 10.

28 Channing, *Treatise*, 18–20.

29 Channing, *Treatise*, 142. Letter printed in the book dated January 22, 1848.

30 Channing, *Treatise*, 147, 149.

31 Channing, *Treatise*, 153.

32 Fuller, *Alternative Medicine and American Religious Life*, 15.

33 Natalie Robins, *Copeland's Cure: Homeopathy and the War between Conventional and Alternative Medicine* (New York: Alfred A. Knopf, 2005), 14–15.

34 Walter Channing, "Address to the Society" in *Boston Medical and Surgical Journal* 62, no. 14 (1860): 387–93; reprinted as pamphlet, in the Rare Book Room of Countway Library of the Harvard Medical School.

35 Fuller, *Alternative Medicine and American Religious Life*, 16.

36 Robins, *Copeland's Cure*, 15.

37 Robins, *Copeland's Cure*, 18.

38 Anton Mesmer (1734–1815) had many teachers, but one was Father Maximillian Hell, a Jesuit priest and astronomer of Vienna who began treating disease in 1770 by using magnetic plates of steel. In 1774 Hell explained his technique to Mesmer, who in turn experimented with the magnetic plates. See Haller, *American Medicine in Transition*, 101.

39 Robins, *Copeland's Cure*, 218.

40 Fuller, *Alternative Medicine and American Religious Life*, 23. See also Madge Pickard and Carlyle Buley, *The Midwest Pioneer: His Ills, Cures, & Doctors* (Crawfordsville, Ind.: Banta, 1945), 15.

41 Haller, *American Medicine in Transition*, 106, 112.

42   Haller, *American Medicine in Transition*, 26–42. See also C. H. G. Jahr, *New Homeopathic Pharmacopoeia and Posology, or the Preparation of Homeopathic Medicines and the Administration of Doses*, trans. James Kitchens (Philadelphia: James Radde, 1842).

43   Fuller, *Alternative Medicine and American Religious Life*. See also *The Water-Cure Journal and Herald of Reforms* 5 (1849).

44   Fuller, *Alternative Medicine and American Religious Life*, 26. See also John A. Brown, *Quackery Exposed!!! Or a few Remarks on the Thomsonian System of Medicine; Consisting of Testimonies and Extracts from Various Writers with Introductory Remarks* (Boston, 1833).

45   Pickard and Buley, *Midwest Pioneer*, 222.

46   Fuller, *Alternative Medicine and American Religious Life*, 33–34.

47   Pickard and Buley, *Midwest Pioneer*, 227.

48   Pickard and Buley, *Midwest Pioneer*, 227.

49   Pickard and Buley, *Midwest Pioneer*, 227.

50   Pickard and Buley, *Midwest Pioneer*, 228.

51   James Ewell, *The Medical Companion, or Family Physician: Treating the Diseases of the United States, with their symptoms, causes, cure and means of prevention: common cases in surgery, as fractures, dislocations &c. the management and diseases of women and children. A dispensatory, for preparing family medicines, and a Glossary explaining technical terms. To which are added a Brief anatomy and Physiology of the human body, showing on rational principles the cause and cure of diseases: An essay on hygiene, or the art of preserving health without the aid of medicine: An American Materia Medica, pointing out the virtues and doses of our medicinal plants also the nurse's guide*, 8th ed. (Philadelphia: Carey, Olea & Blanchard, 1834), xv. See also Mrs. William Parkes, *Domestic Duties* (New York: J & J Harper, 1828), reprinted in a first American edition after having been reprinted twice in London. Parkes's 400-page book is a combination etiquette, household, and marital advice book and includes recipes on cookery, as well as on religion; in the Rare Book Room of Countway Library of the Harvard Medical School.

52   Ewell, *Medical Comparison*, 66–157. See also William Buchan, M.D., *Domestic Medicine; or, a Treatise on the Prevention and Cure of diseases, by Regimen and Simple medicines. With an appendix, containing a dispensatory for the use of private practitioners to which are added Observations on Diet, recommending a method of living less expensive, and more conducive to health than the present. Also, Advice to Mothers, on the subject of their own Health: and of the means of promoting the health, strength, and Beauty of their offspring* (Boston: Joseph Bumstead, 1813); in the Rare Book Room of Countway Library of the Harvard Medical School.

53 Ewell, *Medical Comparison,* 158–59

54 Ewell, *Medical Comparison,* 161–63.

55 Ewell, *Medical Comparison,* 164.

56 Ewell, *Medical Comparison,* 168.

57 Ewell, *Medical Comparison,* 542.

58 Robins, *Copeland's Cure,* 34.

59 Robins, *Copeland's Cure,* 34.

60 Robins, *Copeland's Cure,* 42, 75, 77, 85.

61 David Kirby, *Evidence of Harm: Mercury in Vaccines and the Autism Epidemic: A Medical Controversy* (New York: St. Martin's, 2005).

62 John Marshall, *Remarks on Arsenic, considered as a poison and a medicine; to which are added Five Cases of Recovery from the poisonous effects of arsenic* (London: J. Callow, 1817); in the Rare Book Room of Countway Library of the Harvard Medical School.

63 Kass, *Midwifery and Medicine in Boston,* 137.

64 Badaracco, *Cuba Journal.*

65 Sophia Peabody Hawthorne, 1829 diary, in the Berg Collection of the New York Public Library (hereafter cited simply as the Berg Collection).

66 John H. Winslow, *Darwin's Victorian Malady* (Philadelphia: American Philosophical Society, 1971).

67 Peabody Hawthorne, 1829 diary.

68 Elizabeth Peabody's hand in her sister's 1829 diary, September 3, 1829.

69 Brown, *Quackery Exposed,* 5–8.

70 The other physicians were a Dr. Shattuck, a prominent Bostonian, and Dr. Oliver Hubbard (1772–1842).

71 ALS, Walter Channing to Sophia Peabody, n.d., 1828, in the Berg Collection.

72 ALS, Walter Channing to Sophia Peabody, September 20, 1829, in the Berg Collection.

73 Sophia Peabody, "Dedham Journal," April 11–July 30, 1830, in the Berg Collection.

74 Sophia Peabody, "Dedham Journal," April 11–July 30, 1830, in the Berg Collection.

75 Sophia Peabody, "Boston Journal," January–February 1832, in the Berg Collection.

76 Sophia Peabody, "Boston Journal," January–February 1832, in the Berg Collection.

77 Badaracco, *Cuba Journal.*

78   Badaracco, *Cuba Journal*; ALS Sophia Hawthorne to Annie Adams Fields, January 4, 1866, at Boston Public Library; Sophia Hawthorne to James T. Fields, July 24, 1866; February 25, 1867; June 10, July 7, 1867; January 30, 1868; October 8, 27, November 3, 1867; May 2, 10, 1868, at Boston Public Library.

Chapter 2

1   A10362, Mary Baker Eddy, February 29, 1880, Mary Baker Eddy Collection (hereafter referred to as MBE Collection) [numbers at the beginning of a note are accession numbers for the MBE Collection].

2   Mary Baker Eddy, *Science and Health with Key to the Scriptures* (Boston: First Church of Christ, Scientist, 1994), 143.

3   William A. Purrington, *Christian Science: An Exposition of Mrs. Eddy's Wonderful Discovery, including Legal Aspects A Plea for Children and other Helpless Sick* (New York: E. B. Treat, 1900), 90.

4   Schofield, *Nervousness*, 196.

5   Eddy, *Science and Health*, 144.

6   Eddy, *Science and Health*, 146.

7   Robert Peel, *Christian Science: Its Encounter with American Culture* (New York: Holt, Rinehart & Winston, 1958), 107.

8   J. H. Miller, *Blackwood's* 165 (April 1899): 658–68; *Independent* 67 (October 15, 1909): 888–90; and J. M. Buckley, *North American Review* 173 (July 1901): 22–34.

9   Fuller, *Alternative Medicine and American Religious Life*, 133.

10   Haller, *American Medicine in Transition*, 141.

11   Mary Baker Eddy, *Rudimental Divine Science*, in *Prose Works, Other Than Science and Health* (Boston: W. G. Nixon, 1891), 4.

12   Mary Baker Eddy, "Editor's Table," *Christian Science Journal* (July 1903): 253.

13   Mark Twain, afterword to *Christian Science* (1907; repr. New York: Oxford University Press reprint, 1999), 2.

14   Haller, *American Medicine in Transition*, 141.

15   Gillian Gill, *Mary Baker Eddy*, Radcliffe Biography Series (Reading, Mass.: Perseus, 1998), 88, 68. According to Gill (72), one poem was published in *Godey's Lady's Book*.

16   Gill, *Mary Baker Eddy*, 91.

17   Mary Baker Eddy, *Speaking for Herself* (Boston: Christian Science Board of Directors, 2002), 88–91.

18   Fuller, *Alternative Medicine and American Religious Life*, 59.

19   Eddy, *Speaking for Herself*, 90.

20   Stephen Gottschalk, *Rolling Away the Stone: Mary Baker Eddy's Challenge to Materialism* (Bloomington: Indiana University Press, 2006), 69–70.

21   Gottschalk, *Rolling Away the Stone*, 59–67.

22   A10362, Mary Baker Eddy, February 29, 1880, MBE Collection.

23   VO3343, Mary Baker Patterson to Dr. P. P. Quimby, January 12, 1863, MBE Collection.

24   VO3345, ALS, Mary Baker Patterson to Dr. P. P. Quimby, March 10, 1863, MBE Collection.

25   VO3346, ALS, Mary Baker Patterson to Dr. P. P. Quimby, September 14, 1863, MBE Collection.

26   LO7796, ALS, Mary Baker Patterson to A. G. Dresser, February 15, 1866, MBE Collection.

27   Gill, *Mary Baker Eddy*, 162–63.

28   Gill, *Mary Baker Eddy*, 162–63, citing Mary Baker Eddy, *Retrospection and Introspection*, in *Prose Works, Other Than Science and Health* (Boston: W. G. Nixon, 1891).

29   Eddy, *Speaking for Herself*, 24–25; excerpted from Eddy, *Retrospection and Introspection*.

30   Gottschalk, *Rolling Away the Stone*, 72.

31   A10362, Mary Baker Eddy, February 29, 1880, MBE Collection.

32   Gail M. Harley, *Emma Curtis Hopkins: Forgotten Founder of New Thought* (New York: Syracuse University Press, 2002).

33   Haller, *American Medicine in Transition*, 135n68.

34   A11314, n.d., MBE Collection.

35   In 1916 he was elected as president of the Mother Church. See Yvonne Cache von Fettweis and Robert T. Warneck, *Mary Baker Eddy: Christian Healer* (Boston: Christian Science Association Society, 1998).

36   A11025, article by Mary Baker Eddy, unsigned, n.d., MBE Collection.

37   VO4740, Mary Baker Eddy to editor, n.d., *Boston Post*, 1883.

38   E. J. Arens, *The Understanding of Christianity or God and the Distinction Between Spirit and Matter* (Boston: Alfred Mudge & Sons, 1881). See original pamphlet in Historical File A11553, MBE lawsuits brought. See also James Monroe Buckley, *Faith Healing, Christian Science and Kindred Phenomena* (New York: Century Co., 1892).

39   VO4740, Mary Baker Eddy to editor, *Boston Post*, 1883, MBE Collection.

40   VO4740, Mary Baker Eddy to editor, *Boston Post*, 1883, MBE Collection.

41   LO5498, MBE Collection.

42 Eddy, *Prose Works, Other Than Science and Health* (Boston: W. G. Nixon, 1891), 301.

43 Eddy, *Science and Health*, x.

44 Eddy, *Rudimental Divine Science*, in *Prose Works, Other Than Science and Health* (Boston: W. G. Nixon, 1891), 14–15.

45 EOR21, Calvin Frye, n.d., 1888, MBE Collection.

46 Gill, *Mary Baker Eddy*, 375–78.

47 LO5481, ALS, Mary Baker Eddy to Mary H. Collins, August 30, 1888, MBE Collection; A11560, notes taken in class by Calvin Frye, October 15, 1888, MBE Collection.

48 Gill, *Mary Baker Eddy*, 376.

49 L17011, Typed Letter Signed (TLS), A. Farlow to Mary Baker Eddy, MBE Collection.

50 LO2107, ALS, Mary Baker Eddy to George W. Glover, March 7, 1893, MBE Collection.

51 Von Fettweis and Warneck, *Mary Baker Eddy*.

52 Robert Peel, *Christian Science: Its Encounter with American Culture* (New York: Holt, Rinehart & Winston, 1958), 61, 83.

53 LO6433, TLS, Calvin Frye to Mary Baker Eddy, January 22, 1887, MBE Collection.

54 LO9768, ALS, G. W. Peabody to Mary Baker Eddy, February, 6, 1887, MBE Collection.

55 Christian Science Association, Committee on Publication, letter to the editor of the *Boston Herald*, newsclip dated April 29, 1888. Chestnut Hill files, Historical Collections File, MBE Collection.

56 A10858B, Mary Baker Eddy, typewritten notes for lecture, n.d., MBE Collection.

57 Gill, *Mary Baker Eddy*, 389.

58 Eddy, preface to, *Advice to Healers, Selected Letters*, vol. 3, 1900–1910, MBE Collection.

59 Gill, *Mary Baker Eddy*, 277.

60 Gill, *Mary Baker Eddy*, 287–89.

61 *Boston Globe*, June 4, 1882; see Gill, *Mary Baker Eddy*, 288.

62 Robins, *Copeland's Cure*, 77.

63 William Dana Orcutt, *Mary Baker Eddy and Her Books* (Boston: Christian Science Publication Society, 1950).

64 Longyear Foundation, "Chronology of Physical Changes in Successive Editions of *Science and Health with Key to the Scriptures*, 1875–1911," December 5, 1964; revised October 1966; MBE Research Library.

65 Eddy, entry for creation, in *Key to Scriptures* in *Science and Health*, 238.

66 Orcutt, *Mary Baker Eddy and Her Books*.

67 The word "versus" was interjected between Science and Spiritualism ("and" was deleted); and the word "unmasked" was added, following Animal Magnetism (*Science and Health with Key to Scriptures: Milestones*, typescript, MBE Collection).

68 Gill, *Mary Baker Eddy*, 379.

69 Twain, *Christian Science*, 258.

70 Walter Besant, *The Pen and the Book* (London: Thomas Burleigh, 1899), 153, 155, 156, 160, 177.

71 Besant, *The Pen and the Book*, 207.

72 Judy Huenneke, "MBE and Church Leadership," *Magazine of the MBE Library* 4, no. 4 (2005): 10–16.

73 Christian Science Association minutes, January 2, 1884; see also *Journal of Christian Science*, October 4, 1884; and see *Christian Science Journal*, October 1886 and January 1889.

74 *Journal of Christian Science* 1, no. 1 (April 14, 1883), MBE Collection.

75 "Christian Science Journal 1883–1910 Marketing and Promotion," typescript, MBE Collection.

76 "Christian Science Journal 1883–1910."

77 "Christian Science Journal 1883–1910."

78 *Journal of Christian Science*, October 4, 1884, MBE Collection.

79 TLS, Col. Smith to Mary Baker Eddy, August 19–22, 1885, MBE Collection.

80 "Christian Science Journal 1883–1910."

81 "Christian Science Journal 1883–1910."

82 William G. Nixon to Mary Baker Eddy, October 1888.

83 Joseph Armstrong to MBE, March 13, 1892.

84 Mary Baker Eddy, editorial, *Christian Science Sentinel*, November 30, 1899.

85 Mary Baker Eddy, September 30, 1899.

86 *Christian Science Sentinel* circulation figure, November 30, 1899, MBE Collection.

87 Albert Farlow, see his "Reminiscences," typescript, MBE Collection.

88 Farlow, "Reminiscences," 17.

89 LO1671, A. Farlow to Mary Baker Eddy, October 6, 1904, MBE Collection.

90 LO1671, A. Farlow to Mary Baker Eddy, October 6, 1904, MBE Collection.

91 First Church of Christ, Scientist, Committee on Publication, *Setting the Course: Alfred Farlow and the Mission of the Committee on Publication* (Boston: First Church of Christ, Scientist, 1993).

92 *Setting the Course*, vii.

93 *Setting the Course*, 10.

94 *Setting the Course*, 11. See also Farlow to W. N. Miller, February 27, 1902, MBE Collection.

95 L16780, Farlow to Mary Baker Eddy, TLS, September 19, 1904, MBE Collection.

96 LO9711, TLS, Farlow to Mary Baker Eddy, June 21, 1905, MBE Collection.

97 L16773, Farlow to Mary Baker Eddy, TLS, April 8, 1906, MBE Collection; *Christian Science Journal* (April 8, 1906).

98 *Christian Science Bulletin* (April 11, 1908): 33. See also *Setting the Course*.

99 L16370, TLS, Farlow to Mary Baker Eddy, February 11, 1903, MBE Collection.

100 Willa Cather and Georgine Milmine, *The Life of Mary Baker Eddy and the History of Christian Science* (New York: Doubleday, Page & Co., 1909; repr., Lincoln: University of Nebraska Press, 1993). See also Gottschalk, *Rolling Away the Stone*. The *Christian Science Monitor's* circulation was 60,674 as of March 31, 2006.

101 Erwin D. Canham, *Commitment to Freedom: The Story of the Christian Science Monitor* (New York: Houghton Mifflin, 1958), 58, 60, 65. See also LO7269, Adam H. Dickey to the Board of Trustees of the Christian Science Publishing Company, August 14, 1908, MBE Collection.

102 Canham, *Commitment to Freedom*, 60.

103 Canham, *Commitment to Freedom*, 65.

104 A10646, newsclip, 1889.

105 Canham, *Commitment to Freedom*.

106 Jean A. McDonald, "Mary Baker Eddy at the Podium," (Ph.D. diss., University of Minnesota, 1969), 116.

107 *Chicago Daily Tribune*, June 15, 1888, cited by McDonald, "Mary Baker Eddy," 121.

108 McDonald, "Mary Baker Eddy," 122.

109 Farlow, "Reminiscences," 3–5.

110 A10360A, Mary Baker Eddy sermon, 1878, MBE Collection.

111 *Science and Health*, 135, 141, 159.

112 A10873, scrap 1895, MBE Collection.

113 *Pulpit and Press*, in *Prose Works, Other Than Science and Health* (Boston: W. G. Nixon, 1891), 84.

114 LO8352, TLS, E. Buswell to Mary Baker Eddy, July 12, 1903.

115 LO6986, ALS, Mary Baker Eddy to W. McKenzie, July 20, 1903.

116 A11062, ALS, Mary Baker Eddy to Calvin Frye, August 20, 1905.

117 Bart R. Van Eck, "Spirit versus Matter in Healing," *Christian Science Sentinel*, June 19, 2006, 18. See also www.adherents.com.

118 Rolf Swensen, "Pilgrims at the Golden Gate: Christian Scientists on the Pacific Coast, 1880–1915," *Pacific Historical Review* 72, no. 2 (2003): 229–63, esp. 247.

119 Swensen, "Pilgrims at the Golden Gate," 237, 260, see n68. See also John E. Bauer, *Health Seekers of Southern California, 1870–1900* (San Marino, Calif.: Huntington Library, 1959), 93, 175.

120 Peel, *Christian Science*, 89–90.

121 L12243, TLS, Calvin Frye to Septimus J. Hanna, October 4, 1898, MBE Collection.

122 L14293, TLS, Mary Baker Eddy to F. N. Riale, four lines handwritten by Mary Baker Eddy, September 17, 1906, MBE collection. See also Gottschalk, *Rolling Away the Stone*, 103; LO4171, ALS, Mary Baker Eddy to Emma Lane, March 4, 1888, MBE Collection. Judge Hanna served as editor of Christian Science periodicals 1892–1902, editor of the *Christian Science Journal* in 1891, First Reader in the Mother Church in 1894, was elected president of the church in 1896, and succeeded Mrs. Eddy as president of the Board of Lectureship when she died in 1910, retaining that position until his own death in 1921.

Chapter 3

1 Richard Sloan and Emilia Bagiella, "Data without a Prayer," *Archives of Internal Medicine* 160, no. 12 (2000): 1870; Richard Sloan et al., "Religion, Spirituality and Medicine," *The Lancet* 353, no. 9153 (1999): 664–67; Susan Rhee, Vinod Garg, Charles Hershey, "Use of Complementary and Alternative Medicines by Ambulatory Patients," *Archives of Internal Medicine* 164, no. 9 (2004): 1004–9.

2 Wayne Jonas and Ronald Chez, "Recommendations Regarding Definitions and Standards in Healing Research," *Journal of Alternative and Complementary Medicine* 10, no. 1 (2004): 171–81.

3 Sloan and Bagiella, "Data Without a Prayer"; Jonas and Chez, "Recommendations."

4 Wayne B. Jonas and Cindy C. Crawford, "The Healing Presence: Can It Be Reliably Measured?" *Journal of Alternative and Complementary Medicine* 10, no. 5 (2004): 751–56.

5 Harold Koenig, Michael E. McCullough, and David B. Larson, *Handbook of Religion and Health* (New York: Oxford University Press, 2001); Harold Koenig and Harvey Jay Cohen, eds., *The Link between Religion and Health:*

Psychoneuroimmunology and the Faith Factor (New York: Oxford University Press, 2002)

6   Bruce Rabin, "Understanding How Stress Affects the Body," in *The Link between Religion and Health: Psychoneuroimmunology and the Faith Factor,* ed. Harold Koenig and Harvey Jay Cohen, 43–68, esp. 56–57 (New York: Oxford University Press, 2002).

7   Neal Krause, "Church-Based Social Support and Mortality," *The Journals of Gerontology Series B: Psychological Sciences and Social Sciences* 61 (2006): 140–46. Other studies suggest that rituals, such as eating meals, as well as ethnic prayer influence the health of the elderly. See Brian Buijsse et al., "Cocoa Intake, Blood Pressure, and Cardiovascular Mortality: The Zutphen Elderly Study," *Archives of Internal Medicine* 166, no. 4 (2006): 411–17; Luciano Bernardi et al., "Effect of Rosary Prayer and Yoga Mantras on Autonomic Cardiovascular Rhythms," *British Medical Journal* 323, no. 7327 (2001): 1446–49; also Frank Gillum and Deborah Ingram, "Analysis of the Third National and Nutrition Examination Study, a Multiethnic Sample of 14,500 American Men and Women," *Psychosomatic Medicine* (May/June 2006), released by Reuters, June 13, 2006. The study concluded that people who attended weekly services had lower blood pressure levels than never-attenders.

8   Krause, "Church-Based Social Support"; Anthony Brown, "Religiousness May Lower Blood Pressure in Blacks," Reuters, May 18, 2006, releasing results of the first and presently the only survey of 5,302 African Americans, titled "The Jackson Heart Study," referred to as "the Framingham of the South," referring to the well-known Massachusetts study of a single population cohort.

9   *Health Day* May 5, 2006. See Ronny Bell et al., "Prayer for Health among U.S. Adults: The 2002 National Heath Interview Survey," *Complementary Health Practice Review* 10, no. 3 (2002): 175–88; see also Patricia M. Barnes et al., "Complementary and Alternative Medicine Use among Adults: United States 2002," *Advance Data from Vital and Health Statistics* 343 (May 27, 2004), at http://www.mbcrc.med.ucla.edu/PDFs/camsurvey2 .pdf (accessed May 2, 2007).

10   See Harvard Medical School Web site on Complementary and Alternative Medicine.

11   Anne McCaffrey et al., "Prayer for Health Concerns: Results of a National Survey on Prevalence and Patterns of Use," *Archives of Internal Medicine* 164, no. 8 (2004): 858–62.

12 Steven Strauss, NCCAM *Strategic Plan* (Bethesda, Md.: National Institutes of Health, 2000).

13 Strauss, NCCAM *Stategic Plan.*

14 Jonas and Crawford, "The Healing Presence," 751–75.

15 See also Steven Stumpf and Simon Shapiro, "Bilateral Integrative Medicine, Obviously," *Evidence-Based Complementary and Alternative Medicine* 3, no. 2 (2006): 279–82.

16 Barnes et al., "Complementary and Alternative Medicine Use," http://www.mbcrc.med.ucla.edu/PDFs/camsurvey2.pdf (accessed May 2, 2007).

17 Strauss, NCCAM *Stategic Plan.*

18 Herbert Benson with Marg Stark, *Timeless Healing: The Power and Biology of Belief* (New York: Simon & Schuster, 1996), 234, 239.

19 Jerome Groopman, "No 'Alternative,'" *Wall Street Journal*, August 7, 2006, A12.

20 Groopman, "No 'Alternative.'"

21 Barnes et al., "Complementary and Alternative Medicine Use," http://www.mbcrc.med.ucla.edu/PDFs/camsurvey2.pdf (accessed May 2, 2007).

22 Groopman, "No 'Alternative.'"

23 Rita Agdal, "Diverse and Changing Perceptions of the Body: Communicating Illness, Health, and Risk in an Age of Medical Pluralism," *Journal of Alternative and Complementary Medicine* 11, suppl. 1 (2005): S67–S75.

24 Esther Sternberg, *The Balance Within: The Science Connecting Health and Emotions* (New York: W. H. Freeman, 2001), 169.

25 Harold Koenig, "Clinician's Corner: An 83-Year-Old-Woman with Chronic Illness and Strong Religious Beliefs," *Journal of the American Medical Association* 288, no. 4 (2002): 487–93, esp. 490.

26 An-Fu Hsiao et al., "Variation in Complementary and Alternative Medicine Use Across Racial/Ethnic Groups and the Development of Ethnic-Specific Measures of CAM Use," *Journal of Complementary and Alternative Medicine* 12, no. 3 (2006): 281–90.

27 Hsiao et al., "Variation in Complementary and Alternative Medicine Use," 284.

28 Nobutaka Suzuki, "Complementary and Alternative Medicine: A Japanese Perspective," *Evidenced-based Complementary and Alternative Medicine* 1, no. 2 (2004): 113–18.

29 Randolph C. Byrd, "Positive Therapeutic Effects of Intercessory Prayer in a Coronary Care Unit Population," *Southern Medical Journal* 31 (1988): 826–89.

30 Francis Galton, "Statistical Inquiries into the Efficacy of Prayer," *Fortnightly Review* 12 (1872): 125–35; see also Galton, *Inquiries into Human Faculty and Its Development* (London: Macmillan, 1883).

31 Byrd, "Positive Therapeutic Effects," 826.

32 See C. G. Roland, "Does Prayer Preserve?" *Archives of Internal Medicine* 125 (1970): 580–87, see nn2, 5.

33 Byrd, "Positive Therapeutic Effects," 826.

34 William Harris et al., "A Randomized, Controlled Trial of the Effects of Remote Intercessory Prayer on Outcomes in Patients in Coronary Care Unit," *Archives of Internal Medicine* 159, no. 2 (1999): 273–78.

35 Larry Dossey, "Prayer and Medical Science," *Archives of Internal Medicine* 160, no. 12 (2000): 1735–38, see n7.

36 Willem van der Does, "A Randomized, Controlled Trial of Prayer?" *Archives of Internal Medicine* 160, no. 12 (2000): 1871–72.

37 Jennifer Smith, "The Effect of Remote Intercessry Prayer on Clinical Outcomes," *Archives of Internal Medicine* 160, no. 12 (2000): 1876.

38 Prakash Pande, "Does Prayer Need Testing?" *Archives of Internal Medicine* 160, no. 12 (2000): 1873–74.

39 Sloan and Bagiella, "Data Without a Prayer."

40 Julie Goldstein, "Waiving Informed Consent for Research on Spiritual Matters?" *Archives of Internal Medicine* 160, no. 12 (2000): 1870–71.

41 Dale Hammerschmidt, "Ethical and Practical Problems in Studying Prayer," *Archives of Internal Medicine* 160, no. 12 (2000): 1874–75.

42 Donald Sandweiss, "P Value out of Control," *Archives of Internal Medicine* 160, no. 12 (2000): 1872.

43 Donald Hoover and Joseph Margolick, "Questions on the Design and Findings of a Randomized, Controlled Trial of the Effects of Remote, Intercessory Prayer on Outcomes in Patients Admitted to the Coronary Care Unit," *Archives of Internal Medicine* 160, no. 12 (2000): 1875–76.

44 Fred Rosner, "Therapeutic Efficacy of Prayer," *Archives of Internal Medicine* 160, no. 2 (2000): 1875.

45 Mitchel Galishoff et al., "God, Prayer, and Coronary Unit Outcomes: Faith vs. Works," *Archives of Internal Medicine* 160, no. 12 (2000): 1877.

46 Raymond F. Palmer, David Katerndahl, and Jayne Morgan-Kidd, "A Randomized Trial of the Effects of Remote Intercessory Prayer: Interactions with Personal Beliefs on Problem-Specific Outcomes and Functional Status," *Journal of Alternative and Complementary Medicine* 10, no. 3 (2004): 438–48.

47 Palmer et al., "Randomized Trial."

48   Benson and Stark, *Timeless Healing*,

49   Brian Bolton, "God, Science and Intercessory Prayer," *Journal of Alternative and Complementary Medicine* 162, no. 12 (2004): 1422–23.

50   J. T. Chibnall et al., "Experiments on Distant Intercessory Prayer," *Journal of Internal Medicine* 161 (2001): 2529–36; Jeffrey Bishop, "Retroactive Prayer: Lots of History, Not Much Mystery, and No Science," *British Medical Journal* 329 (2004): 1444–46; Jeffrey Bishop, "Prayer, Science, and the Moral Life of Medicine," *Archives of Internal Medicine* 163, no. 12 (2003): 1405–8.

51   Jonas and Crawford, "The Healing Presence."

52   Herbert Benson et al., "Study of the Therapeutic Effects of Intercessory Prayer (STEP) in Cardiac Bypass Patients: A Multicenter Randomized Trial of Uncertainty and Certainty of Receiving Intercessory Prayer," *American Heart Journal* 151, no. 4 (2006): 934–42.

53   Drew Leder, "Spooky Actions at a Distance: Physics, Psi and Distant Healing," *Journal of Alternative and Complementary Medicine* 11, no. 5 (2005): 923–30.

54   Benson at al., "STEP in Cardiac Bypass Patients," 935.

55   Mitchell Krucoff, Suzanne Crater, and Kerry Lee, "From Efficacy to Safety Concerns: A STEP Forward or a Step Back for Clinical Research and Intercessory Prayer? The Study of Therapeutic Effects of Intercessory Prayer (STEP)," *American Heart Journal* 151, no. 4 (2006): 762–64.

56   Benson et al., "STEP in Cardiac Bypass Patients," 941, 942.

57   Krucoff, Crater, and Lee, "From Efficacy to Safety Concerns," 763.

58   Jeffery Dusek et al., "Study of the Therapeutic Effects of Intercessory Prayer (STEP): Study Design and Research Methods," *American Heart Journal* 143, no. 4 (2001): 577–84; Benson et al., "STEP in Cardiac Bypass Patients," 933.

59   Jeanne Achterberg et al., "Evidence for Correlations between Distant Intentionality and Brain Function in Recipients: A Functional Magnetic Resonance Imaging Analysis," *Journal of Alternative and Complementary Medicine* 11, no. 6 (2005): 965–71.

60   Wayne Jonas and Cindy Crawford, eds., *Healing Intention and Energy Medicine: Science, Research Methods and Clinical Implications* (New York: Churchill Livingstone, 2003).

61   Jonas and Crawford, "The Healing Presence."

62   Herbert Benson with Miriam Z. Klipper, *The Relaxation Response* (New York: Quill/Harper Collins, 2001).

63   Achterberg et al., "Evidence for Correlations," 968, 970.

64 Wayne Jonas, "The Middle Way: Realistic Randomized Controlled Trials for the Evaluation of Spiritual Healing," *Journal of Alternative and Complementary Medicine* 7, no. 1 (2001): 5–7.

65 Koenig, McCullough, and Larson, *Handbook of Religion and Health*, 36–37.

66 Peter Hill and Ralph Hood, *Measure of Religiosity* (Birmingham, Ala.: Religious Education Press, 1999), 212; and Bruce Rabin and Harold Koenig, "Immune, Neuroendocrine, and Religious Measures," in *The Link between Religion and Health: Psychoneuroimmunology and the Faith Factor*, ed. Harold Koenig and Harvey Jay Cohen, 197–249 (New York: Oxford University Press, 2002).

67 Rabin and Koenig, "Immune, Neuroendocrine, and Religious Measures," 212.

68 Harold Koenig, "Integrative Medicine: Integrating Conventional and Alternative Medicine; The Journal of Integrative Medicine," *Journal of the American Medical Association* 283, no. 22 (2000): 2993–94.

69 Rabin and Koenig, "Immune, Neuroendocrine, and Religious Measures," 212, 223.

70 Rabin and Koenig, "Immune, Neuroendocrine, and Religious Measures," 220–23.

71 See G. W. Allport and J. M. Ross, "Personal Religious Orientation and Pre-judice," *Journal of Personality and Social Psychology* 5 (1967): 432–43.

72 Rabin and Koenig, "Immune, Neuroendocrine, and Religious Measures," 223.

73 Fetzer Institute. Kalamazoo, Michigan.

74 Rabin and Koenig, "Immune, Neuroendocrine, and Religious Measures," 224.

75 Paul Griffiths, "Psychoneuroimmunology and Eastern Religions Traditions," in *The Link between Religion and Health: Psychoneuroimmunology and the Faith Factor*, ed. Harold Koenig and Harvey Jay Cohen, 250–61 (New York: Oxford University Press, 2002).

76 Dalai Lama, *Ethics for the New Millenium* (New York: Riverhead Books, 1999).

77 Warren S. Brown, "Psychoneuroimmunology and Western Religious Traditions," in *The Link between Religion and Health: Psychoneuroimmunology and the Faith Factor*, ed. Harold Koenig and Harvey Jay Cohen, 262–74 (New York: Oxford University Press, 2002).

78 Timothy Daaleman, "Religion, Spirituality, and the Practice of Medicine," *Journal of the American Board of Family Medicine* 17, no. 5 (2004): 370–76.

79 Brown, "Psychoneuroimmunology," 262.

80 Howard L. Kaye, "Psychoneuroimmunology and Religion: Implications for Society and Culture," in *The Link between Religion and Health: Psychoneuroimmunology and the Faith Factor*, ed. Harold Koenig and Harvey Jay Cohen, 275–85 (New York: Oxford University Press, 2002).

81 Sloan and Begiella, "Data Without a Prayer;" Jonas and Crawford, "Healing Presence."

82 Bishop, "Prayer, Science, and the Moral Life of Medicine," 1405–8.

Chapter 4

1   Ralph Snyderman, lecture presented at the "Investigating the Mind 2005: Science and Clinical Applications of Meditation" conference, November 8–10, 2005, Washington, D.C. DVD, *Investigating the Mind 2005: The Science and Clinical Applications of Meditation*. Mind and Life series 12 (Washington, D.C.: Mind and Life Institute, 2005).

2   Eddy, *Science and Health*.

3   Pema Chödrön, *When Things Fall Apart* (Boston: Shamhala, 2002), 52; Thich Nhat Hanh, *Being Peace* (Berkeley, Calif.: Parallax, 1987), 3.

4   Thomas Merton, *Mystics and Zen Masters* (New York: Farrar, Straus & Giroux, 1967), 202–5.

5   Thomas Merton, *What Is Contemplation* (New York: Templegate, 1950), 50.

6   Thomas Merton, *Life and Holiness* (New York: Herder & Herder, 1963), 50.

7   Abraham Joshua Heschel, ed., *I Asked for Wonder: A Spiritual Anthology* (New York: Crossroad, 2001), 32.

8   McCaffrey et al., "Prayer for Health Concerns: Results of a National Survey on Prevalence and Patterns of Use," 858–62.

9   McCaffrey et al., "Prayer for Health Concerns: Results of a National Survey on Prevalence and Patterns of Use," 858–62.

10 McCaffrey et al., "Prayer for Health Concerns: Results of a National Survey on Prevalence and Patterns of Use," 858–62.

11 E. A. Mayer and C. B. Saper, eds., *The Biological Basis for Mind-Body Interactions*, Progress in Brain Research 122 (New York: Elsevier, 2000).

12 NCCAM Web site; N. Mikhail, S. Wali, and I. Ziment, "Use of Alternative Medicine among Hispanics," *Journal of Alternative and Complementary Medicine* 10, no. 5 (2004): 851–59.

13 Herbert Benson and Jeff Dusek, "Self-Reported Health, and Illness and the Use of Conventional and Unconventional Medicine and Mind/Body Healing by Christian Scientists and Others," *Journal of Nervous and Mental Disease* 187, no. 9 (1999): 539–48.

14   Benson and Dusek, "Self-Reported Health."

15   Joel Schulman and Keith Maedor, *Heal Thyself: Spirituality, Medicine, and the Distortion of Christianity* (New York: Oxford University Press, 2003).

16   Case Western Reserve Medical School's Center for the Study of Unlimited Love is conducting research on altruism, optimism, and positive thinking.

17   Mayer and Saper, *The Biological Basis for Mind-Body Interactions.*

18   George F. Solomon, "The Development and History of Psychoneuroimmunology," in *The Link between Religion and Health: Psychoneuroimmunology and the Faith Factor*, ed. Harold Koenig and Harvey Jay Cohen, 31–43, esp. 33 (New York: Oxford University Press, 2002).

19   Solomon, "The Development and History of Psychoneuroimmunology," 33.

20   Esther Sternberg, *The Balance Within* (New York: W. H. Freeman, 2001); Bruce McEwen, "Protective and Damaging Effects of Stress Mediators: Central Role of the Brain," in *The Biological Basis for Mind-Body Interactions*, Progress in Brain Research 122, ed. E. A. Mayer and C. B. Saper, 25 (New York: Elsevier, 2000).

21   Sternberg, *The Balance Within*, 35, 36, 61.

22   McEwen, "Protective and Damaging Effects."

23   Barnes et al., "Complementary and Alternative Medicine Use," http://www.mbcrc.med.ucla.edu/PDFs/camsurvey2.pdf (accessed May 2, 2007).

24   Bruce Rabin, "Understanding How Stress Affects the Body," in *The Link between Religion and Health: Psychoneuroimmunology and the Faith Factor*, ed. Harold Koenig and Harvey Jay Cohen, 43–68 (New York: Oxford University Press, 2002).

25   Richard L. Verrier and Murray A. Mittleman, "The Impact of Emotions on the Heart," in *The Biological Basis for Mind-Body Interactions*, ed. E. A. Mayer and C. B. Saper, Progress in Brain Research 122, 370–78 (New York: Elsevier, 2000).

26   Benson and Klipper, *The Relaxation Response*; Herbert Benson with William Proctor, *Beyond the Relaxation Response* (New York: Times Books, 1984); and Herbert Benson, *Timeless Healing: The Power and Biology of Belief* (New York: Scribner, 1996).

27   The author attended several sessions at Harvard Medical School's Mind Body Medicine Institute between 2005–2006.

28   Nhat Hanh, *Being Peace*, x.

29   Jon Kabat-Zinn, lecture presented at the "Investigating the Mind 2005: Science and Clinical Applications of Meditation" conference, November 8–10, 2005, Washington, D.C. DVD, *Investigating the Mind 2005: The Science and Clinical Applications of Meditation*. Mind and Life series 12 (Washington,

D.C.: Mind and Life Institute, 2005), Dr. Kabat-Zinn's Stress Reduction Clinic is located at the University of Massachusetts Medical Center, Amherst.

30 Mathieu Ricard, lecture presented at the "Investigating the Mind 2005: Science and Clinical Applications of Meditation" conference, November 8–10, 2005, Washington, D.C. DVD, *Investigating the Mind 2005: The Science and Clinical Applications of Meditation*. Mind and Life series 12 (Washington, D.C.: Mind and Life Institute, 2005).

31 Ricard, lecture at "Investigating the Mind 2005."

32 Dalai Lama, *Ethics for the New Millenium*, 161–81.

33 Ricard, lecture at "Investigating the Mind 2005."

34 Ajahn Amaro, lecture presented at the "Investigating the Mind 2005: Science and Clinical Applications of Meditation" conference, November 8–10, 2005, Washington, D.C. DVD, *Investigating the Mind 2005: The Science and Clinical Applications of Meditation*. Mind and Life series 12 (Washington, D.C.: Mind and Life Institute, 2005).

35 Pema Chödrön, *When Things Fall Apart*.

36 Nhat Hanh, *Being Peace*.

37 Thomas Merton, *Seeds of Contemplation* (1949; repr., New York: New Directions, 1986).

38 Kabat-Zinn, lecture at "Investigating the Mind 2005."

39 Richard Davidson, lecture presented at the "Investigating the Mind 2005: Science and Clinical Applications of Meditation" conference, November 8–10, 2005, Washington, D.C. DVD, *Investigating the Mind 2005: The Science and Clinical Applications of Meditation*. Mind and Life series 12 (Washington, D.C.: Mind and Life Institute, 2005).

40 Zindel V. Segal, lecture presented at the "Investigating the Mind 2005: Science and Clinical Applications of Meditation" conference, November 8–10, 2005, Washington, D.C. DVD, *Investigating the Mind 2005: The Science and Clinical Applications of Meditation*. Mind and Life series 12 (Washington, D.C.: Mind and Life Institute, 2005).

41 Segal, lecture at "Investigating the Mind 2005."

42 B. Alan Wallace, lecture presented at the "Investigating the Mind 2005: Science and Clinical Applications of Meditation" conference, November 8–10, 2005, Washington, D.C. DVD, *Investigating the Mind 2005: The Science and Clinical Applications of Meditation*. Mind and Life series 12 (Washington, D.C.: Mind and Life Institute, 2005). See also B. Alan Wallace, *Contemplative Science: Where Buddhism and Neuroscience Converge* (New York: Columbia University Press, 2007).

43   Snyderman, lecture at "Investigating the Mind 2005."

44   Snyderman, lecture at "Investigating the Mind 2005."

45   Jeffrey Bishop, "Prayer, Science, and the Moral Life of Medicine."

46   N. Schoenberger et al., "Opinions and Practices of Medical Rehabilitation Professionals Regarding Prayer and Meditation," *Journal of Alternative and Complementary Medicine* 8, no. 1 (2002): 59–69.

47   Harold Koenig, "Clinician's Corner," *Journal of the American Medical Association* 288, no. 4 (2002): 487–93.

48   Farr A. Curlin et al., "The Association of Physicians' Religious Characteristics With Their Attitudes and Self-Reported Behaviors Regarding Religion and Spirituality in the Clinical Encounter," *Medical Care* 44, no 5 (2006): 446–53.

49   Koenig, "Clinician's Corner," 491.

50   Stefan Schmidt, "Mindfulness and Healing Intention: Concepts, Practice, and Research Evaluation," *Journal of Alternative and Complementary Medicine* 10, suppl. 1 (2004): S7–S14.

51   Schmidt, "Mindfulness and Healing Intention."

52   Schmidt, "Mindfulness and Healing Intention," S8.

53   Schmidt, "Mindfulness and Healing Intention."

54   Schmidt, "Mindfulness and Healing Intention," S9.

55   Schmidt, "Mindfulness and Healing Intention."

56   Schmidt, "Mindfulness and Healing Intention."

57   Frederic Luskin, " Transformative Practices for Integrating Mind Body Spirit," *Journal of Alternative and Complementary Medicine* 10, suppl. 1 (2004): S15–23, esp. S19.

58   Marc Kaufman, "Dalai Lama Speaks to Scientists," *Washington Post*, November 9, 2005.

59   Kaufman, "Dalai Lama Speaks to Scientists."

60   Tenzin Gyatso, the Dalai Lama, "Science at the Crossroads," November 12, 2005. Mind and Life Institute, http://www.mindandlife.org/dalai.lama .sfndc.html (accessed May 7, 2007).

61   Dalai Lama, "Science at the Crossroads."

62   Dalai Lama, *Ethics for the New Millennium*.

63   Dalai Lama, *Ethics for the New Millennium*.

64   Schulman and Maedor, *Heal Thyself*, 91.

65   Schulman and Maedor, *Heal Thyself*, 91.

66   Schulman and Maedor, *Heal Thyself*, 92.

67   Schulman and Maedor, *Heal Thyself*, 94.

68   Schulman and Maedor, *Heal Thyself*, 94.

69 Benson uses professional writers to help reach mass publics. See chapter 4, n26 for his coauthors.

70 See Herbert Benson, "Yoga for Drug Abuse," *New England Journal of Medicine* 281, no. 20 (1969): 1133; and Benson with R. K. Wallace, "Decreased Drug Abuse with Transcendental Meditation—A Study of 1,862 Subjects," in *Drug Abuse—Proceedings of the International Conference*, ed. Chris J. D. Zarafonetis, 369–376 (Philadelphia: Lea & Febiger, 1972); Herbert Benson, "Transcendental Meditation—Science or Cult?" *Journal of the American Medical Association* 227, no. 7 (1974): 807.

71 Benson, *Relaxation Response.*

Chapter 5

1 The concept discussed by Richard John Neuhaus in, *The Naked Public Square: Religion and Democracy in America*, 2nd ed. (Grand Rapids: Eerdmans, 1986).

2 Amaro, lecture at "Investigating the Mind 2005"; Howard Wolinsky, "Disease Mongering and Drug Marketing," *Science and Society* (EMBO reports) 6, no. 7 (2005); Greg Crister, *Generation RX: How Prescription Drugs Are Altering American Lives, Minds and Bodies* (New York: Houghton Mifflin, 2005), 134. See also Lynn Payer, *Disease-Mongers: How Doctors, Drug Companies, and Insurers Are Making You Feel Sick*, (New York: John Wiley & Sons, 1992). Payer was the first medical journalist to develop the nomenclature for identifying this trend. Moynihan and Cassels, Crister and Angell all advance her theory with additional evidence. See also Bob Burton and Andy Rowell, "Disease Mongering," Center for Media and Democracy, http://www.prwatch.org/prwissues/2003Q1/monger.html (accessed June 14, 2007).

3 Crister, *Generation RX*, 222; See also Sofia Ahmed et al., "Gender Bias in Cardiovascular Advertisements," *Journal of Evaluation in Clinical Practice* 4, no. 10 (2005): 531–38.

4 Craig Aaron, Taylor Lincoln, and Neal Pattison, *The Other Drug War 2003: Drug Companies Deploy an Army of 675 Lobbyists to Protect Profits* (Washington, D.C.: Public Citizen's Congress Watch, June 2003); cited in Marcia Angell, *The Truth about the Drug Companies: How They Deceive Us and What to Do about It* (New York: Random House, 2005); John F. Kamp, "Citizen Petition Requesting Promulgation of an Amended Regulation for Prescription Drug Advertising to Establish Separate Criteria for Practitioner-Directed and Consumer-Directed Advertising and to Establish a Standing Advisory Committee on Health Care Communications"

(Rockville, Md.: Coalition for Healthcare Communication, 2006), http://www.cohealthcom.org/content/FinalCHCCitizenPetition.pdf (accessed May 8, 2007).

5   Angell, *The Truth about the Drug Companies*; see also Ray Moynihan and Alan Cassels, *Selling Sickness: How the World's Biggest Pharmaceutical Companies are Turning Us All into Patients* (New York: Avalon, 2005). See also Crister, *Generation RX*.

6   The phrase "branded condition" is from Vincent Parry, U.K. advertising executive. See the video, *Selling Sickness: An Ill for Every Pill*, directed by Catherine Scott, produced by Pat Fiske (Brooklyn, N.Y.: Icarus Films, 2004); Leonore Tiefer, "Female Sexual Dysfunction: A Case Study of Disease Mongering and Activist Resistance," *PLoS Medicine* 3, no. 4/e178 (2006): 0436–40, http://medicine.plosjournals.org/archive/1549-1676/3/4/pdf/10.1371_journal.pmed.0030178-L.pdf (accessed May 8, 2007).

7   Robins, *Copeland's Cure*. Angell, *The Truth about Drug Companies*, 179. See also Andy Kessler, *The End of Medicine: How Silicon Valley (and Naked Mice) . . . will Reboot Your Doctor* (New York: Collins, 2006).

8   Moynihan and Cassels, *Selling Sickness*, and Parry in Scott, *Selling Sickness*. See also National Institutes of Health, "News from the Women's Health Initiative: Reducing Total Fat Intake May Have Small Effect on Risk of Breast Cancer, No Effect on Risk of Colorectal Cancer, Heart Disease, or Stroke," press release, February 7, 2006, http://www.nih.gov/news/pr/feb2006/nhlbi-07.htm (accessed May 8, 2007); and three complete articles on these findings in the *Journal of the American Medical Association* 295, no. 6 (2006): 629–66.

9   Crister, *Generation RX*, 134; Parry in Scott, *Selling Sickness*; Benson, *Relaxation Response*; The FDA attitude toward direct-to-consumer advertising is uncritical. For two examples, see Tamar Nordenberg, "Direct to You: TV Drug Ads That Make Sense," *FDA Consumer Magazine* (January–February 1998): 1–4, http://www.fda.gov/fdac/features/1998/198_ads.html (accessed May 8, 2007). More recently, see Carol Rados, "Truth in Advertising: RxDrugs Ads Come of Age," *FDA Consumer Magazine* (July–August 2004), http://www.fda.gov/fdac/features/2004/404_ads.html (accessed May 8, 2007), in which she argues, "There seems to be little doubt that DTC advertising can help advance the public health by encouraging more people to talk with health care professionals about health problems, particularly under-treated conditions such as high blood pressure and high cholesterol"; reprinted in John E. Richardson, ed.,

Business Ethics 06/07, Contemporary Learning Series 18th ed (Dubuque, IA: McGraw-Hill, 2007).

10 Elizabeth Almasi et al., "What Are the Public Health Effects of DTC Drug Advertising?" *PLoS Medicine* 3, no. 3/e145 (2006): 0284–88.

11 Crister, *Generation RX*, 222; for a contrary view, see John E. Calfee, Clifford Winston, and Randolph Stempski, "Direct-to-Consumer Advertising and the Demand for Cholesterol-Reducing Drugs," *Journal of Law and Economics* 45, no. 2/2 (2002): 673–90; also available through AEI-Brookings Joint Center for Regulatory Studies, as Related Publication 03-12, June 2003, http://www.aei-brookings.org/admin/authorpdfs/page.php?id=269 (accessed May 8, 2007); for a business perspective see Charles Hunt, *Interaction of Detailing and Journal Advertising: How Detailing and Journal Advertising Impact New Prescriptions* (New York: Association of Medical Publications, 2005), http://www.rxpromoroi.org/pdf/interaction_whitepaper.pdf (accessed May 8, 2007).

12 K. Aiken, "Patient and Physician Attitude and Behaviors Associated with DTC Promotion of Prescription Drugs—Summary of FDA Survey Research Results," November 14, 2004; U.S. Department of Health and Human Services, "Guidance for Industry: Consumer-Directed Broadcast Advertisements," August 1999, http://www.fda.gov/cber/gdlns/advrts.pdf (accessed May 8, 2007); American Medical Association, on Consumer Directed Promotion, docket No. 2003N-0344, http://www.fda.gov/OHRMS/DOCKETS/dailys/03/dec03/120303/03N-0344-emc-000020-01.pdf (accessed May 8, 2007); Margaret Gilhooley, FDA Docket No. 2005N- 0354, February 16, 2006, "Comments on Consumer-Directed Promotion of Regulated Medical Products," http://www.fda.gov/OHRMS/DOCKETS/dockets/05n0354/05N-0354-EC437-Attach-1.pdf (accessed May 8, 2007). See also Angell, *The Truth about the Drug Companies*; Crister, *Generation RX*; Moynihan and Cassels, *Selling Sickness*.

13 Angell, *The Truth about the Drug Companies*.

14 Jacky Law, *Big Pharma: Exposing the Global Healthcare Agenda* (New York: Carroll & Graf, 2006).

15 PhRMA, press release, August 2, 2005.

16 Crister, *Generation RX*, 133; Federal Trade Commission, "FTC Proposes Study of Competitive Impact of Authorized Generic Drugs," press release, March 29, 2006; Federal Trade Commission, "FTC Charges Bristol-Myers Squibb with Pattern of Abusing Government Processes to Stifle Generic Drug Competition: Alleged Illegal Conduct Involves Three

Drugs, Includes Improper Orange Book Listings and Unlawful Agreements in Restraint of Trade," press release, March 7, 2006.

17 Angell, *The Truth about the Drug Companies*, 173. Authors of the bill were Orrin Hatch, R-Utah, and Henry Waxman, D-Calif; see Federal Trade Commission, "FTC Recommends Legislative Changes to Hatch-Waxman Act," press release, July 30, 2002, http://www.ftc.gov/opa/2002/07/genericdrugstudy.shtm (accessed May 8, 2007).

18 PhRMA, 2005 Annual Report, 2–4. In 2005, PhRMA invested $51.3 billion in biopharameutical research and development: in Phase I, $9.6 billion; Phases II–III, $15.9 billion, and close to another $8 billion for producing the "strong evidence of safety," plus ongoing studies of drug safety required by the FDA.

19 Angell, *The Truth about the Drug Companies*, 174–78.

20 Angell, *The Truth about the Drug Companies*, 174–78; see also Food and Drug Administration, "Prescription Drug Marketing Act Pedigree Requirements; Effective Date and Compliance Policy Guide; Request for Comment," *Federal Register* 71, no. 114 (2006): 34249.

21 Jeanne Whalen, "How Glaxo Marketed a Malady to Sell a Drug: TV-Ad Blitz, Physician Onslaught Are Unleashed to Inform about Little-Known Disorder," *Wall Street Journal*, October 26, 2006, B2; Leonard Weber, *Profits before People: Ethical Standards and Marketing of Prescription Drugs* (Bloomington: Indiana University Press, 2006), 157–81.

22 Whalen, "How Glaxo"; Steven Woloshin and Lisa Schwartz, "Giving Legs to Restless Legs: A Case Study of How the Media Helps Make People Sick," *PLoS Medicine* 3, no. 4/e170 (2006): 0452–55. See also Judy Illes et al., "Advertising, Patient Decision Making and Self-referral for Computed Tomographic and Magnetic Resonance Imaging," *JAMA Archives of Internal Medicine* 164, no. 22 (2004): 2415–19.

23 Woloshin and Schwartz, "Giving Legs to Restless Legs."

24 Joanna Breitstein, "The Making of a New Disease," *Pharmaceutical Executive* (January 1, 2004): 1–8, http://www.pharmexec.com/pharmexec/article/articleDetail.jsp?id=80917 (accessed May 8, 2007). Naming the syndrome, a link between obesity, diabetes, and hypertension, was the work of German researchers in the late 1970s, revived by Gerald Reaven, a Stanford University professor in 1988, citing "insulin resistance" as the link between a person's normal level of pancreatic secretion and those whose levels were too low to "unlock glucose" from food and transport it to the body's cells for energy.

25 Breitstein, "The Making of a New Disease"; see also Annabel Ferriman, "Novartis Breached Code after Doctors Say it 'Invented a Disease,'" *British Medical Journal* 325 (December 14, 2002): 1379, http://www.bmj.com/cgi/reprint/325/7377/1379.pdf (accessed May 8, 2007).

26 Breitstein, "The Making of a New Disease," 4.

27 Breitstein, "The Making of a New Disease," 2.

28 PhRMA, 2005 Annual Report, 4; PhRMA, press release, September 29, 2005, testimony before Congress of the PhRMA Chief Medical Officer Paul Antony, on DTC Guidelines; press release, August 2, 2005, speech by CEO Billy Tauzin to the American Legislative Exchange 32nd Annual Meeting on Guiding Principles of DTC Advertising, approved on July 29, 2005, went into effect January 2006.

29 PhRMA, 2005 Annual Report. See also Charles Smith and James O'Donnell, *The Process of New Drug Discovery and Development* (Boca Raton, Fla.: Taylor & Francis, 2006).

30 Breitstein, "The Making of a New Disease," 7.

31 Al Ries and Laura Ries, *The Fall of Advertising and the Rise of PR* (New York: Harper Business, 1994).

32 Heather Tesoriero, "Merck Suffers Vioxx Case Setbacks," *Wall Street Journal*, August 18, 2006, A2; Alex Berenson, "Merck Suffers a Pair of Setbacks over Vioxx," *New York Times*, August 18, 2006, C1; Peter Loftus, "Merck's Vioxx Tied to New Threat; Heart Risks Start Early in Study," *Wall Street Journal*, September 13, 2006, A12.

33 Associated Press report, in *Wall Street Journal*, July 13, 2006, D7.

34 Gina Kolata, "Drug for Bones Is Linked to Jaw Disease," *New York Times*, June 2, 2006, A17; Jennifer Dooren, "Restrictions Curb Use of Powerful Acne Drug," *Wall Street Journal*, September 12, 2006, D1–D4. Accutane is one of four isotretinoin drugs available, and is reported as highly effective against serious acne that can cause disfigurement. The drug is so powerful that among the birth defects it can cause are misshapen heads, missing ears, and heart defects. Because the FDA requires everyone taking the drug to register for it and to see a dermatologist monthly to get a renewal, people are turning to the Internet for illegal prescriptions. Reportedly two hundred women a year get pregnant while taking the drug. See also Michael R. Albert and Kristen G. Ostheimer, "The Evolution of Current Medical and Popular Attitudes toward Ultraviolet Light Exposure: Part 3," *Journal of the American Academy of Dermatology* 49, no. 6 (2003): 1096–1106.

35 *Wall Street Journal,* July 28, 2006, A3.

36 Roddy Boyd, "Pfizer's Pflap," *New York Post,* June 8, 2006, 41; Melody Petersen, "Pfizer Settles an Inquiry into Ads for an Antibiotic," *New York Times,* January 7, 2003, C7.

37 Patrick Clinton, "Phase Six: Regain Confidence," *Pharmaceutical Executive* (April 1, 2005): 1, http://www.pharmexec.com/pharmexec/article/article Detail.jsp?id=162120 (accessed May 8, 2007). Vos cites a book by David Maister, Charles Green, and Robert Galford, *Trusted Advisor* (New York: Free Press, 2000).

38 Burton and Rowell, "Disease Mongering"; see also Erica Goode, "Antidepressants Lift Clouds, but Lose 'Miracle Drug' Label," *New York Times,* June 30, 2002, A1.

39 Clinton, "Phase Six." See also Diana Kohnle, "Cancer Drug Ads Put Caveats in Fine Print," *HealthDay,* June 7, 2006, http://www.healthday .com/Article.asp?AID=533122 (accessed May 8, 2007), who cites a study presented to the American Society of Clinical Oncology done by Dr. Gregory Abel of ads in three magazines for the year 2005 directed to cancer patients. Abel concludes from his study that the language of clinical trials, while suitable for the clinical encounter with a cancer patient, is inappropriate for advertising because it is difficult to read.

40 Clinton, "Phase Six." See also, as an example of CAM treatment, Joel Finkelstein, "Calcium Plus Vitamin D for Postmenopausal Women—Bone Appetit?" *New England Journal of Medicine* 354, no. 7 (2006): 750–52.

41 Clinton, "Phase Six."

42 Clinton, "Phase Six," 2.

43 Clinton, "Phase Six," 5.

44 Clinton, "Phase Six," 6.

45 Interview with Don Apruzzese, "Drug Companies Stir Emotions to Draw Attention," *Pharmaceutical Executive* (July 1, 2006): 1–3.

46 Barbara Mintzes, "Disease Mongering in Drug Promotion: Do Governments Have a Regulatory Role," *PLoS Medicine* 3, no. 4/e198 (2006): 0461–65, http://medicine.plosjournals.org/archive/1549-1676/3/4/pdf/10.1371_journal.pmed.0030198-L.pdf (accessed May 8, 2007).

47 Mintzes, "Disease Mongering," 0462n19, citing a Merck Web site accessed in 2006.

48 Mintzes, "Disease Mongering"; see also Ray Moynihan, "The Marketing of a Disease: Female Sexual Dysfunction," *British Medical Journal* 330, no. 7484 (2005): 192–95.

49   Clinton, "Phase Six"; see also the correction, "Error in Financial Disclosure in Conjugated Equine Estrogens and Coronary Heart Disease: The Women's Health Initiative," *Archives of Internal Medicine* 166, no. 7 (2006): 759; this correction refers back to an article in the February 13 issue of *Archives of Internal Medicine* 166, no. 3 (2006): 357–65.

50   See Crister, *Generation RX*; Angell, *The Truth about the Drug Companies*; Moynihan and Cassels, *Selling Sickness*; and Law, *Big Pharma*; see also R. A. Hansen et al., "Factors Influencing the Shift of Patients from One Proton Pump Inhibitor to Another: The Effect of Direct-to-Consumer Advertising," *Clinical Therapeutics* 27, no. 9 (2005): 1478–87.

51   Gardiner Harris, "Report Finds a Heavy Toll from Medication Errors," *New York Times*, July 21, 2006, A12.

52   See Crister, *Generation RX*; Angell, *The Truth about the Drug Companies*; Moynihan and Cassels, *Selling Sickness*; and Law, *Big Pharma*.

53   Crister, *Generation RX*, 140–66.

54   Crister, *Generation RX*, 140.

55   A. Harmon, "Young, Assured and Playing Pharmacist to Friends," *New York Times*, November 16, 2005, A1, A18.

56   Crister, *Generation RX*, 145.

57   Crister, *Generation RX*, 77.

58   Moynihan, and Cassels, *Selling Sickness*, 4.

59   Crister, *Generation RX*, 77.

60   Moynihan, and Cassels, *Selling Sickness*.

61   Crister, *Generation RX*, 163.

62   Crister, *Generation RX*, 221.

63   Angell, *The Truth about the Drug Companies*.

64   Crister, *Generation RX*, 102; see also P. Cathebras, "Doctor Knock Lives at Wall St.: The New Targets of the Pharmaceutical Industry," *Revue de Medecine Interne* 24, no. 8 (2003): 538–41 (in French).

65   Crister, *Generation RX*, 114.

66   Crister, *Generation RX*, 145.

67   Moynihan and Cassels, *Selling Sickness*, 4, ix.

68   Crister, *Generation RX*, 119.

69   Crister, *Generation RX*, 114; Moynihan and Cassels, *Selling Sickness*, 4. CHAD has more than 15,000 members in more than 200 affiliates.

70   N. W. Read, "Bridging the Gap between Mind and Body: Do Cultural and Psychoanalytic Concepts of Visceral Disease Have an Explanation in Contemporary Neuroscience?" in *The Biological Basis for Mind-Body*

Interactions, Progress in Brain Research 122, ed. E. A. Mayer and C. B. Saper, 427 (New York: Elsevier, 2000).

71   Moynihan and Cassels, *Selling Sickness*.

72   J. Coe, *Healthcare: The Lifestyle Drug Outlook to 2008, Unlocking New Value in Well-Being* (Reuters Business Insight, 2003); cited by Moynihan and Cassels, *Selling Sickness*, 4.

73   Moynihan and Cassels, *Selling Sickness*, 63.

74   Crister, *Generation RX*, 163.

75   Angell, *The Truth about the Drug Companies*. See also Crister, *Generation RX*, 221; Moynihan and Cassels, *Selling Sickness*, 89.

76   Angell, *The Truth about the Drug Companies*.

77   David Armstrong, "Medical Journal Editor Nemeroff Steps Down over Undisclosed Ties," *Wall Street Journal*, August 28, 2006, B7.

78   Reed Abelson, "Charities Tied to Doctors Get Drug Industry Gifts," *New York Times*, June 28, 2006, A1, C4.

79   David Armstrong, "Aspirin Dispute Is Fueled by Funds Of Industry Rivals," *Wall Street Journal*, April 24, 2006, A1, A12.

80   Melody Petersen, "Madison Ave. Has Growing Role in the Business of Drug Research," *New York Times*, November 22, 2002, A1. See also Whalen, "How Glaxo Marketed a Malady."

81   Crister, *Generation RX*, 123.

82   Moynihan and Cassels, *Selling Sickness*, 42; Brian Steinberg, "TV's Pauley Sues *New York Times*," *Wall Street Journal*, October 27, 2006, B5.

83   Crister, *Generation RX*, 117.

84   Crister, *Generation RX*, 121.

85   Robert Steinbrook, "For Sale: Physicians' Prescribing Data," *The New England Journal of Medicine* 354, no. 26 (2006): 2745–47.

86   Steinbrook, "For Sale"; Crister, *Generation RX*, 121. According to Crister, the AMA now gives physicians the right to block access to sales representatives, while permitting other officials or pharmaceutical corporations full access. New Hamphire banned the sale and use of data in which prescribers are identified; presumably other states will follow. Data would be available for "noncommercial use," grouping the doctors by zip code, specialty, and geography, but not listing their names, providing just the end-run that PR practitioners need.

87   Crister, *Generation RX*, 118; Angell, *The Truth about the Drug Companies*, 121.

88   See Moynihan and Cassels, *Selling Sickness*; Angell, *The Truth about Drug Companies*; Crister, *Generation RX*; and NCCAM Web site.

89   Angell, *The Truth about the Drug Companies*, 48, 120.

90   Mintzes, "Disease Mongering in Drug Promotion", Angell, *The Truth about the Drug Companies*, 120–24; see also Tiefer, "Female Sexual Disfunction."

91   "Drug Makers Raise Ad Spending," *Wall Street Journal*, October 6, 2006, B4. Until 1997, full disclosure of side effects and risks was required, but since the list of side effects were too long to include in a thirty-second or sixty-second ad or in a print advertisement, modifications were made after pressure by industry. Since 1997, the FDA regulations are satisfied by a shorter version of the side effects, limited to key copy points and mention of where the consumer can read further information on the Internet. If the advertisement is judged to be unfairly representing the product, the agency is supposed to send a warning letter, after it is reviewed by its legal office and the matter is listed on the FDA Web site.

92   Mintzes, "Disease Mongering in Drug Promotion," see 0464, table 1. See also, M. Rosenthal, "Comment: The Economics of Direct-to-Consumer Advertising of Prescription-only Drugs: Prescribed to Improve Consumer Welfare?" *Journal of Health Services Research and Policy* 9, no. 1 (2004): 39–42.

93   Amanda Gardner, "Experts Fault New FDA Drug Label Changes," *Health-Day*, June 7, 2006, http://www.healthday.com/Article.asp?AID=533155 (accessed May 8, 2007).

94   Jerry Avorn and William Shrank, "Highlights and a Hidden Hazard— The FDA's New Labeling Regulations," *New England Journal of Medicine* 354, no. 23 (2006): 2409–11.

95   Ann Wilde Mathews, "Rising FDA Reliance on 'User Fees' Boosts Drug Firms' Clout in Talks," Infinite Health Resources, January 1, 2007, online, http://www.infinitehealthresources.com/Store/Resource/Article/1-10-86/3/1077.html (accessed May 8, 2007).

96   Mintzes, "Disease Mongering in Drug Promotion."

97   Mathews, "Rising FDA Reliance."

98   According to Nader's report, PhRMA employed 112 lobbyists at a cost of $14.3 million. The top ten drug companies and trade associations spent $55.8 million, accounting for more than half the amount spent on lobbying industry-wide. Brand-name drug manufacturers spent $76 million to lobby their cause, compared to the measly $3.4 million spent by generic drug manufacturers.

99   PhRMA, 2005 Annual Report, 22; PhRMA Report: "Medicines in Development for Neurologic Disorders," 2006.

100 Mariana Maggini, Nicola Vanacore, and Roberto Raschetti, "Cholinesterase Inhibitors: Drugs Looking for a Disease?" *PLoS Medicine* 3, no. 4/e140

(2006): 0456–60, http://medicine.plosjournals.org/archive/1549-1676/3/4/pdf/10.1371_journal.pmed.0030140-L.pdf (accessed May 8, 2007).

101 Kalman Applbaum, "Pharmaceutical Marketing and the Invention of the Medical Consumer," *PLoS Medicine* 3, no. 4/e189 (2006): 0445–47, http://medicine.plosjournals.org/archive/1549-1676/3/4/pdf/10.1371_journal.pmed.0030189-L.pdf (accessed May 8, 2007).

Conclusion

1 William James, *The Varieties of Religious Experience: A Study in Human Nature* (New York: Modern Library, 2002 edition).

2 Amanda Gardner, "U.S. Panel Endorses Cervical Cancer Vaccine for Girls," *HealthDay*, June 29, 2006, http://healthday.com/Article.asp?AID=533557 (accessed May 8, 2007); Amanda Gardner, "FDA Approves Cervical Cancer Vaccine," *HealthDay* June 8, 2006, http://healthday.com/Article.asp?AID=533156 (accessed May 8, 2007); Marc K. Siegel, "Polarized Pills," *New York Post*, June 23, 2006.

3 Institute of Medicine, "Report Brief—The Future of Drug Safety: Action Steps for Congress," (Washington, D.C.: National Academies Press, September 2006), http://www.iom.edu/Object.File/Master/37/331/11750_report_brief_congress.pdf (accessed May 8, 2007).

4 Jay Tolson, "Is There Room for the Soul? New Challenges to Our Most Cherished Beliefs about Self and the Human Spirit," *US News & World Report*, October 23, 2006, 57–63. http://www.usnews.com/usnews/health/articles/061015/23soul_3.htm (accessed May 8, 2007).

SELECTED READINGS

Alcott, A. Bronson. *Conversation with Children about the Gospels.* Boston: J. Monroe, 1836.

Almasi, Elizabeth, et al., "What Are the Public Health Effects of DTC Drug Advertising?" *PLoS Medicine* 3, no. 3/e145 (2006).

Angell, Marcia. *The Truth about the Drug Companies: How They Deceive Us and What to Do about It.* New York: Random House, 2005.

Applbaum, Kalman. "Pharmaceutical Marketing and the Invention of the Medical Consumer." *PLoS Medicine* 3, no. 4/e189 (2006): 1–10.

Aaron, Craig, Taylor Lincoln, and Neal Pattison, *The Other Drug War 2003: Drug Companies Deploy an Army of 675 Lobbyists to Protect Profits.* Congress Watch, June 2003. Washington, D.C.: Public Citizen, 2003.

Badaracco, Claire. *American Culture and the Marketplace.* Washington, D.C.: Center for the Book, Library of Congress, 1993.

———. *The Cuba Journal, 1833–35, of Sophia Peabody Hawthorne.* From the Holograph in the Berg Collection of the New York Public Library. UMI Press, Books on Demand, 1982.

———. "Pitfalls and Rewards of the Solo Editor: Sophia Peabody Hawthorne." *Resources in American Literary Studies* 11, no. 1 (1980): 91–100.

————. *Trading Words*. Baltimore: Johns Hopkins University Press, 1995.

Badaracco, Claire, ed. *Quoting God: How Media Shape Ideas about Religion*. Waco, Tex.: Baylor University Press, 2005.

Barnes, Linda, and Susan Sered, eds. *Religion and Healing in America*. New York: Oxford University Press, 2006.

Benson, Herbert. *Beyond the Relaxation Response*. New York: Penguin, 1984.

————. "Decreased Drug Abuse with Transcendental Meditation—A Study of 1,862 Subjects." In *Drug Abuse—Proceedings of the International Conference*, edited by C. J. D. Zarafonetis, 369–76. Philadelphia: Lea & Febiger, 1972.

————. *Timeless Healing: The Power and Biology of Belief*. New York: Fireside/Simon & Schuster, 1996.

————. "Transcendental Meditation—Science or Cult?" *Journal of the American Medical Association* 227, no. 7 (1974): 807.

————. "Yoga for Drug Abuse." *New England Journal of Medicine* 281, no. 20 (1969): 1133.

Benson, Herbert, et al. "Study of the Therapeutic Effects of Intercessory Prayer (STEP) in Cardiac Bypass Patients: A Multicenter Randomized Trial of Uncertainty and Certainty of Receiving Intercessory Prayer." *American Heart Journal* 151, no. 4 (2006): 934–42.

Benson, Herbert, and Jeff Dusek. "Self-Reported Health, and Illness and the Use of Conventional and Unconventional Medicine and Mind/Body Healing by Christian Scientists and Others," *Journal of Nervous and Mental Disease* 187, no. 9 (1999): 539–48.

Benson, Herbert, with Marg Stark. *Timeless Healing: The Power and Biology of Belief*. New York: Simon & Schuster, 1996.

Besant, Walter. *The Pen and the Book*. London: Thomas Burleigh, 1899.

Bloom, Harold. *The American Religion*. New York: Simon & Schuster, 1992.

Buckley, James Monroe. *Faith Healing, Christian Science and Kindred Phenomena*. New York: Century Co., 1892.

Burton, Bob, and Andy Rowell. "Disease Mongering." *North American Animal Liberation Press Office Newsletter* 1, no. 4 (2004): 35–39. http://animalliberationfront.com/News/NAALPO/newsletter_V1no4_0905.pdf (accessed May 7, 2007).

Calfee, John E., Clifford Winston, and Randolph Stempski. "Direct-to-Consumer Advertising and the Demand for Cholesterol-Reducing

Drugs." *Journal of Law and Economics* 45, no. 2/2 (2002): 673–90. Reissued through AEI-Brookings Joint Center for Regulatory Studies, as Related Publication 03-12, June 2003. http://www.aei-brookings.org/admin/authorpdfs/page.php?id=269 (accessed May 8, 2007).

Canham, Erwin D. *Commitment to Freedom: the Story of the Christian Science Monitor.* New York: Houghton Mifflin, 1958.

Cather, Willa, and Georgine Milmine. *The Life of Mary Baker Eddy and the History of Christian Science.* New York: Doubleday, Page & Co., 1909. Reprint, Lincoln: University of Nebraska Press, 1993.

Channing, Walter. Review of John Elwell, *A Medico-Legal Treatise on Malpractice and Medical Evidence, Comprising the Elements of Medical Jurisprudence.* Boston Medical and Surgical Journal 62, no. 12 (April 19, 1860): 233–41.

———. *A Treatise on Etherization in Childbirth Illustrated by Five Hundred and Eighty-one Cases.* Boston: Ticknor & Fields, 1848.

Chödrön, Pema. *When Things Fall Apart.* Boston: Shambhala, 2002.

Cohen, Michael H. *Healing at the Borderland of Medicine and Religion.* Chapel Hill: University of North Carolina Press, 2006.

Crister, Greg. *Generation RX: How Prescription Drugs Are Altering American Lives, Minds and Bodies.* New York: Houghton Mifflin, 2005.

Dalai Lama (TenzinGyatso). "Science at the Crossroads." Speech to the Annual Meeting of the Association of Neuroscientists, 2005.

Douglas, Ann. *The Feminization of American Culture.* New York: Alfred Knopf, 1977.

Ewell, James. *The Medical Companion, or Family Physician.* 8th edition. Philadelphia: Carey, Olea & Blanchard, 1834.

Fuller, Robert. *Alternative Medicine and American Religious Life.* New York: Oxford University Press, 1989.

Gill, Gillian. *Mary Baker Eddy.* Radcliffe Biography Series. Reading, Mass.: Perseus, 1998.

Gottschalk, Stephen. *Rolling Away the Stone: Mary Baker Eddy's Challenge to Materialism.* Bloomington: Indiana University Press, 2006.

Haller, John S. *American Medicine in Transition, 1840–1910.* Urbana: University of Illinois Press, 1981.

Harley, Gail. *Emma Curtis Hopkins: Forgotten Founder of New Thought.* Syracuse, N.Y.: Syracuse University Press, 2002.

Hershock, Peter. *Reinventing the Wheel: A Buddhist Response to the Informa-tion Age.* Albany: State University Press of New York, 1999.

Heschel, Abraham Joshua, ed. *I Asked for Wonder: A Spiritual Anthology.* New York: Crossroad, 2001.

Holmes, Oliver Wendell. "Border Lines of Knowledge in Some Provinces of Medical Science: An Introductory Lecture, Delivered before the Medical Class of Harvard University, November 6, 1861." Boston: Ticknor & Fields, 1862.

————. *Medical Essays, 1842–1882.* 1883; repr., Boston: Houghton, Mif-flin, 1891.

————. *Puerperal Fever as a Private Pestilence.* Boston: Ticknor & Fields, 1855.

Hoover, Stewart, and Knut Lundby. *Rethinking Media, Religion and Culture.* Thousand Oaks, Calif.: Sage, 1997.

Hoover, Stewart, and Lynn Clark, eds. *Practicing Religion in the Age of the Media.* New York: Columbia University Press, 2002.

Institute of Medicine. *The Future of Drug Safety: Promoting and Protecting the Health of the Public.* Report Brief, September 2006. Washington, D.C.: National Academies Press, 2006.

Jeffrey, David Lyle. *People of the Book: Christian Identity and Literary Cul-ture.* Grand Rapids: Eerdmans, 1996.

Jonas, Wayne, and Ronald Chez. "Recommendations Regarding Defi-nitions and Standards in Healing Research." *Journal of Alternative and Complementary Medicine* 10, no. 1 (2004): 171–81.

Jonas, Wayne, and Cindy Crawford. "The Healing Presence: Can It Be Reliably Measured?" *Journal of Alternative and Complementary Medicine* 10, no. 5 (2004): 751–75.

Kass, Amalie. *Midwifery and Medicine in Boston: Walter Channing, M.D., 1786–1876.* Boston: Northeastern University Press, 2002.

Khema, Ayya. *Be an Island: The Buddhist Practice of Inner Peace.* Boston: Wisdom Publications, 1999.

Kirby, David. *Evidence of Harm: Mercury in Vaccines and the Autism Epi-demic: A Medical Controversy.* New York: St. Martin's Press, 2005.

Koenig, Harold G. *Faith and Mental Health: Religious Resources for Healing.* Philadelphia: Templeton Foundation Press, 2005.

Koenig, Harold G., and Harvey Jay Cohen, eds. *The Link between Reli-gion and Health: Psychoneuroimmunology and the Faith Factor.* New York: Oxford University Press, 2002.

Koenig, Harold G., with Gregg Lewis. *The Healing Connection: The Story of a Physicians Search for the Link between Faith and Health*. Philadelphia: Templeton Foundation Press, 2004.

Koenig, Harold G., Michael E. McCullough, and David B. Larson. *Handbook of Religion and Health*. New York: Oxford University Press, 2001.

Law, Jacky. *Big Pharma: Exposing the Global Healthcare Agenda*. New York: Carroll & Graf, 2006.

Lovallo, William. *Stress and Health: Biological and Psychological Interactions*. Thousand Oaks, Calif.: Sage, 1997.

Marshall, Megan. *The Peabody Sisters*. Boston: Houghton Mifflin, 2005.

Merton, Thomas. *Mystics and Zen Masters*. New York: Farrar, Straus & Giroux, 1967.

Miller, William R., and John E. Martin. *Behavior Therapy and Religion: Integrating Spiritual and Behavioral Approaches to Change*. Newbury Park, Calif.: Sage, 1988.

Mind and Life Institute. *Investigating the Mind 2005: The Science and Clinical Applications of Meditation*. Mind and Life series 12. Washington, D.C.: Mind and Life Institute, 2005.

Mintzes, Barbara. "Disease Mongering in Drug Promotion: Do Governments Have a Regulatory Role?" *PLoS Medicine* 3, no. 4/e198 (2006): 0461–65.

Mitchell, Jolyon, and Sophia Marriage, eds. *Mediating Religion: Conversations in Media, Religion and Culture*. London: T&T Clark, 2003.

Moynihan, Ray. 2005. "The Marketing of a Disease: Female Sexual Dysfunction." *British Medical Journal* 330, no. 7484 (2005): 192–95

Moynihan, Ray and Alan Cassels. *Selling Sickness: How the World's Biggest Pharmaceutical Companies Are Turning Us All into Patients*. New York: Avalon Nation Books, 2005.

Newberg, Andrew B., Eugene G. D'Aquili, and Vince Rause. *Why God Won't Go Away: Brain Science and the Biology of Belief*. New York: Ballantine, 2001.

Nhat Hanh, Thich. *Being Peace*. Berkeley, Calif.: Parallax, 1997.

Nord, David. *Faith in Reading: Religious Publishing and the Birth of Mass Media in America*. New York: Oxford University Press, 2004.

Nordenberg, Tamar. "Direct to You: TV Drug Ads That Make Sense." *FDA Consumer Magazine* (January–February 2004): 1–4.

Ohmann, Richard. *Selling Culture: Magazines, Markets, and Class at the Turn of the Century.* New York: Verso, 1996.

Orcutt, William Dana. *Mary Baker Eddy and Her Books.* Boston: Christian Science Publication Society, 1950.

Payer, Lynn. *Disease-Mongers: How Doctors, Drug Companies, and Insurers Are Making You Feel Sick.* New York: John Wiley & Sons, 1992.

Peabody, Elizabeth Palmer. 1880. "Female Education in Massachusetts." *Barnard's American Journal of Education* 30 (1880): 584.

———. *Record of a School: Exemplifying the General Principles of Spiritual Culture.* Boston: J. Monroe, 1835.

Peel, Robert. *Christian Science: Its Encounter with American Culture.* New York: Holt, Rinehart & Winston, 1958.

Purrington, William. *Christian Science: An Exposition of Mrs. Eddy's Wonderful Discovery, including Legal Aspects. A Plea for Children and Other Helpless Sick.* New York: E. B. Treat, 1900.

Robins, Natalie. *Copeland's Cure: Homeopathy and the War between Conventional and Alternative Medicine.* New York: Alfred A. Knopf, 2005.

Schulman, Joel, and Keith Maedor. *Heal Thyself: Spirituality, Medicine, and the Distortion of Christianity.* New York: Oxford University Press, 2003.

Scott, Catherine. *Selling Sickness: An Ill for Every Pill.* Brooklyn, N.Y.: Icarus Films, 2004.

Steinbrook, Robert. "For Sale: Physicians' Prescribing Data." *New England Journal of Medicine* 354, no. 26 (2006): 2745–47.

Sternberg, Esther. *The Balance Within: The Science Connecting Health and Emotions.* New York: W. H. Freeman, 2001.

Stevenson, Scott. *Famous Illnesses in History.* London: Eyrie & Spottiswoode, 1962.

Stout, Daniel, and Judith Buddenbaum. *Religion and Popular Culture: Studies on the Interaction of Worldviews.* Ames: Iowa State University Press, 2001.

Tiefer, Leonore. "Female Sexual Dysfunction: A Case Study of Disease Mongering and Activist Resistance." *PLoS Medicine* 3, no. 4/e178 (2006): 0436–40.

Twain, Mark. *Christian Science.* New York: Harper & Bros., 1907; repr. New York: Oxford University Press reprint, 1999.

Twitchell, James. *Branded Nation*. New York: Simon & Schuster, 2004.

Verrier, Richard L., and Murray A. Mittleman, "The Impact of Emotions on the Heart." In *The Biological Basis for Mind-Body Interactions*. Edited by E. A. Mayer and C. B. Saper. Progress in Brain Research 122, 370–78. New York: Elsevier, 2000.

Wallace, B. Allan. *Contemplative Science: Where Buddhism and Neuroscience Converge*. New York: Columbia University Press, 2007.

Weber, Leonard. *Profits before People: Ethical Standards and Marketing of Prescription Drugs*. Bloomington: Indiana University Press, 2006.

Winslow, John. *Darwin's Victorian Malady*. Philadelphia: American Philosophical Society, 1971.

Woody, Thomas. *A History of Women's Education in the U.S.* New York: Octagon, 1929.

INDEX

Abbot, Abiel, 44
Abbott, Lyman, 54
Abbott Laboratories, 182
abortion, 23, 66, 100, 120
Accumetrics, Inc., 187–88
Accutane, 176, 236n34
acid reflux, 160, 182
acquired immunodeficiency
    syndrome (AIDS), 100, 102
acupuncture, 99, 103
Adderall, 185
The Adventures of Huckleberry Finn
    (Twain), 75–76
advertising
    American cultural attitudes,
        199–202
    books and mass media, 201–02
    Christian Science publications,
        76–79, 82–83
    as consumer education, 156–59,
        162, 236n39

direct-to-consumer, 166, 169–70,
    175–78, 183, 191–92, 206–07,
    232n9
ethics of, 35–36, 165–66
medical advice in, 151–54
prescription drug, 72–73, 185–89
research journal publishing, 185–86
side effects and risks, 239n91
user fees, 192–93
See also mass media;
    pharmaceutical industry
African Americans, 222n8
Agassiz, Louis, 54
aging and cognitive impairment
    creating a disease of, 156, 196
    pharmaceutical industry and,
        194–96
    predisease development, 182
    "sandwich generation" and, 165
alcohol, 19, 28–29, 159, 206
Alcott, A. Bronson, 29, 44–45, 53, 87